W9-BNA-044

Birth Control

**Recent Titles in
Q&A Health Guides**

Birth Control

Your Questions Answered

Paul Quinn

Q&A Health Guides

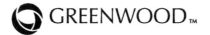

GREENWOOD™

An Imprint of ABC-CLIO, LLC
Santa Barbara, California • Denver, Colorado

Library of Congress Cataloging-in-Publication Data

Names: Quinn, Paul, 1971– author.
Title: Birth control : your questions answered / Paul Quinn.
Description: Santa Barbara, CA : Greenwood, an imprint of ABC-CLIO, LLC, [2019] |
    Series: Q&A health guides | Includes bibliographical references and index.
Identifiers: LCCN 2018051691 (print) | LCCN 2018053152 (ebook) |
    ISBN 9781440862717 (ebook) | ISBN 9781440862700 (print : alk. paper)
Subjects: LCSH: Birth control. | Youth—Sexual behavior.
Classification: LCC HQ766 (ebook) | LCC HQ766 .Q85 2019 (print) |
    DDC 613.9—dc23
LC record available at https://lccn.loc.gov/2018051691

ISBN: 978-1-4408-6270-0 (print)

    978-1-4408-6271-7 (ebook)

23 22 21 20 19   1 2 3 4 5

This book is also available as an eBook.

Greenwood
An Imprint of ABC-CLIO, LLC

ABC-CLIO, LLC
147 Castilian Drive
Santa Barbara, California 93117
www.abc-clio.com

This book is printed on acid-free paper ∞

Manufactured in the United States of America

This book discusses treatments (including types of medication and mental health therapies), diagnostic tests for various symptoms and mental health disorders, and organizations. The authors have made every effort to present accurate and up-to-date information. However, the information in this book is not intended to recommend or endorse particular treatments or organizations, or substitute for the care or medical advice of a qualified health professional, or used to alter any medical therapy without a medical doctor's advice. Specific situations may require specific therapeutic approaches not included in this book. For those reasons, we recommend that readers follow the advice of qualified health care professionals directly involved in their care. Readers who suspect they may have specific medical problems should consult a physician about any suggestions made in this book.

For Mom and David . . . once again

Contents

Series Foreword

All of us have questions about our health. Is this normal? Should I be doing something differently? Whom should I talk to about my concerns? And our modern world is full of answers. Thanks to the Internet, there's a wealth of information at our fingertips, from forums where people can share their personal experiences to Wikipedia articles to the full text of medical studies. But finding the right information can be an intimidating and difficult task—some sources are written at too high a level, others have been oversimplified, while still others are heavily biased or simply inaccurate.

Q&A Health Guides address the needs of readers who want accurate, concise answers to their health questions, authored by reputable and objective experts, and written in clear and easy-to-understand language. This series focuses on the topics that matter most to young adult readers, including various aspects of physical and emotional well-being as well as other components of a healthy lifestyle. These guides will also serve as a valuable tool for parents, school counselors, and others who may need to answer teens' health questions.

All books in the series follow the same format to make finding information quick and easy. Each volume begins with an essay on health literacy and why it is so important when it comes to gathering and evaluating health information. Next, the top five myths and misconceptions that surround the topic are dispelled. The heart of each guide is a collection of questions and answers, organized thematically. A selection of five case studies provides real-world examples to illuminate key concepts. Rounding out each volume are a directory of resources, glossary, and index.

It is our hope that the books in this series will not only provide valuable information but also help guide readers toward a lifetime of healthy decision making.

Acknowledgments

This work would not be possible without the support and encouragement from my family, friends, and colleagues. Specifically, sincere thanks and appreciation to Eileen Guidice, David Gilsenan, "Maggie and Milo," Tina Neri-Badame, Gregory Locoparra, Denise Mojica, Mary Quinn, Kelly Greco, Joe and Gail Guidice, Anthony and Laura Guidice, Roxanne Guidice, Donna Petrolia, John and Mindy Gilsenan, Mike and Mary Lanni, Christine Lanni, Michael Lanni and Alyssa DeJoy, John and Gina Nicoletti-Gilsenan, Kate and Marwan Amaisse, Matt Gilsenan, and the memory of Gladys Gilsenan. In addition, Robert Velez, Maryanne Hedrick, Larry Lane, Joel Kunkel and Chris Vano, Jim McCoy, Sean and Marie Sherrock, Ian Klein, Felipe Guzman, Marvin Kasper, Ann Marie Leichman, Charles Vannoy, Peter Jarosz and my friends, and coworkers and colleagues of The Valley Health System were a constant source of support and encouragement.

I remain extremely grateful to Maxine Taylor, Lettie Conrad, and Tracey Molineaux for their literary, publishing, and promotional expertise and direction.

Some people never get to meet their heroes or guardian angel—I was raised with mine. Thank you, Vinny, for the spirit that pushes me to do more and be more than I ever imagined.

Finally, I can do this work only because of the invaluable lessons I have learned from the men and women I have had the honor to care for, my patients—for over two decades of nursing and midwifery practice. Your lives, stories, resilience, and spirit are forever part of my soul.

Introduction

Over 50 percent of the pregnancies in the United States are unplanned, with 3 million women becoming pregnant unintentionally each year. However, the use of some form of contraception continues to increase along with the number of men and women who are purposely opting to be sexually active but avoiding the possibility of pregnancy. According to the U.S. Center for Disease Control and Prevention, 62 percent of women in the United States are currently using some form of contraception, demonstrating that the use of birth control, or contraception, is rising. The scientific community and the pharmaceutical industry have addressed the increased need for specialized, safe methods of contraception. However, the number of options for both men and women has become staggering and can often be confusing when attempting to choose which method will best serve an individual or couple.

Education has been highlighted as a key strategy to assist an individual or couple to choose which contraceptive method or option would work best for them. A plethora of information exists on the Internet and in print regarding the various birth control methods. Anyone can search a specific method and review its pros and cons or read other people's experiences with their use of a specific method. In addition, birth control has become popularized through television commercials or print advertisements in major magazines or newspapers. However, the information contained on specific websites or in commercially available public information can be misleading or biased. Not all the information on the Internet or in print is factual, accurate, or applicable for all men or women. Further, the risks, complications, side effects, or impact on future fertility are often absent or ignored. Birth control, however, is not for everyone. There is also a wide variation among the existing birth control methods. Some methods, for example, purposely require a prescription, while others can be purchased over the counter. Overall, each method of birth control is safe when it is selected and used properly and consistently by an individual.

The objective of this book is to break down the stigma surrounding the use of birth control and discuss the various options currently available for men, women, or couples to choose from when deciding on birth control. By providing information and education in a simple format regarding each of the various types or forms of birth control, their mechanism of action, contraindications, benefits, risks, use, side effects, complications, and their impact on a return to fertility, this book answers important, common questions people have regarding the use of birth control, or contraception. Further, this book can be used to develop questions for individuals to ask their health-care practitioner when exploring their birth control options. Sex and sexual activity carry no shame; however, irresponsible, unprotected sex or sexual activity can have deleterious outcomes for an individual or couple. Informed, responsible decision-making prevents an individual, or couple, from being impacted by the consequences of an unplanned pregnancy. Birth control is individualized and comprehensive to each individual or couple. The evolution of birth control over the past three decades has allowed an open, honest dialog regarding contraception to occur and has led to the development of safer birth control options. This book answers the questions many people are afraid, or embarrassed, to ask using the most recent, accurate, scientific evidence available in easy-to-understand language.

Guide to Health Literacy

On her 13th birthday, Samantha was diagnosed with type 2 diabetes. She consulted her mom and her aunt, both of whom also have type 2 diabetes, and decided to go with their strategy of managing diabetes by taking insulin. As a result of participating in an after-school program at her middle school that focused on health literacy, she learned that she can help manage the level of glucose in her bloodstream by counting her carbohydrate intake, following a diabetic diet, and exercising regularly. But, what exactly should she do? How does she keep track of her carbohydrate intake? What is a diabetic diet? How long should she exercise, and what type of exercise should she do? Samantha is a visual learner, so she turned to her favorite source of media, YouTube, to answer these questions. She found videos from individuals around the world sharing their experiences and tips, doctors (or at least people who have "Dr." in their YouTube channel names), government agencies such as the National Institutes of Health, and even video clips from cat lovers who have cats with diabetes. With guidance from the librarian and the health and science teachers at her school, she assessed the credibility of the information in these videos and even compared their suggestions to some of the print resources that she was able to find at her school library. Now, she knows exactly how to count her carbohydrate level, how to prepare and follow a diabetic diet, and how much (and what) exercise is needed daily. She intends to share her findings with her mom and her aunt, and now she wants to create a chart that summarizes what she has learned that she can share with her doctor.

Samantha's experience is not unique. She represents a shift in our society; an individual no longer views himself or herself as a passive recipient of medical care but as an active mediator of his or her own health. However, in this era when any individual can post his or her opinions and experiences with a particular health condition online with just a few clicks or publish a memoir, it is vital that people know how to assess the credibility of health information. Gone are the days when "publishing" health information required intense vetting. The health information landscape is highly saturated, and people have innumerable sources where they can find information about practically any health topic. The sources (whether print, online, or a person) that an individual consults for health information are crucial because the accuracy and trustworthiness of the information can potentially affect his or her overall health. The ability to find, select, assess, and use health information constitutes a type of literacy—health literacy—that everyone must possess.

THE DEFINITION AND PHASES OF HEALTH LITERACY

One of the most popular definitions for health literacy comes from Ratzan and Parker (2000), who describe health literacy as "the degree to which individuals have the capacity to obtain, process, and understand basic health information and services needed to make appropriate health decisions." Recent research has extrapolated health literacy into health literacy bits, further shedding light on the multiple phases and literacy practices that are embedded within the multifaceted concept of health literacy. Although this research has focused primarily on online health information seeking, these health literacy bits are needed to successfully navigate both print and online sources. There are six phases of health information seeking: (1) Information Need Identification and Question Formulation, (2) Information Search, (3) Information Comprehension, (4) Information Assessment, (5) Information Management, and (6) Information Use.

The first phase is the *information need identification and question formulation phase.* In this phase, one needs to be able to develop and refine a range of questions to frame one's search and understand relevant health terms. In the second phase, *information search,* one has to possess appropriate searching skills, such as using proper keywords and correct spelling in search terms, especially when using search engines and databases.

It is also crucial to understand how search engines work (i.e., how search results are derived, what the order of the search results means, how to use the snippets that are provided in the search results list to select websites, and how to determine which listings are ads on a search engine results page). One also has to limit reliance on surface characteristics, such as the design of a website or a book (a website or book that appears to have a lot of information or looks aesthetically pleasant does not necessarily mean it has good information) and language used (a website or book that utilizes jargon, the keywords that one used to conduct the search, or the word "information" does not necessarily indicate it will have good information). The next phase is *information comprehension*, whereby one needs to have the ability to read, comprehend, and recall the information (including textual, numerical, and visual content) one has located from the books and/or online resources.

To assess the credibility of health information (*information assessment* phase), one needs to be able to evaluate information for accuracy, evaluate how current the information is (e.g., when a website was last updated or when a book was published), and evaluate the creators of the source—for example, examine site sponsors or type of sites (.com, .gov, .edu, or .org) or the author of a book (practicing doctor, a celebrity doctor, a patient of a specific disease, etc.) to determine the believability of the person/organization providing the information. Such credibility perceptions tend to become generalized, so they must be frequently reexamined (e.g., the belief that a specific news agency always has credible health information needs continuous vetting). One also needs to evaluate the credibility of the medium (e.g., television, Internet, radio, social media, and book) and evaluate—not just accept without questioning—others' claims regarding the validity of a site, book, or other specific source of information. At this stage, one has to "make sense of information gathered from diverse sources by identifying misconceptions, main and supporting ideas, conflicting information, point of view, and biases" (American Association of School Librarians [AASL], 2009, p. 13) and conclude which sources/information are valid and accurate by using conscious strategies rather than simply using intuitive judgments or "rules of thumb." This phase is the most challenging segment of health information seeking and serves as a determinant of success (or lack thereof) in the information-seeking process. The following section on Sources of Health Information further explains this phase.

The fifth phase is *information management*, whereby one has to organize information that has been gathered in some manner to ensure easy retrieval and use in the future. The last phase is *information use*, in which one will synthesize information found across various resources, draw conclusions, and locate the answer to his or her original question and/or the content that fulfills the information need. This phase also often involves implementation, such as using the information to solve a health problem; make health-related decisions; identify and engage in behaviors that will help a person to avoid health risks; share the health information found with family members and friends who may benefit from it; and advocate more broadly for personal, family, or community health.

THE IMPORTANCE OF HEALTH LITERACY

The conception of health has moved from a passive view (someone is either well or ill) to one that is more active and process based (someone is working toward preventing or managing disease). Hence, the dominant focus has shifted from doctors and treatments to patients and prevention, resulting in the need to strengthen our ability and confidence (as patients and consumers of health care) to look for, assess, understand, manage, share, adapt, and use health-related information. An individual's health literacy level has been found to predict his or her health status better than age, race, educational attainment, employment status, and income level (National Network of Libraries of Medicine, 2013). Greater health literacy also enables individuals to better communicate with health care providers such as doctors, nutritionists, and therapists, as they can pose more relevant, informed, and useful questions to health care providers. Another added advantage of greater health literacy is better information-seeking skills, not only for health but also in other domains, such as completing assignments for school.

SOURCES OF HEALTH INFORMATION: THE GOOD, THE BAD, AND THE IN-BETWEEN

For generations, doctors, nurses, nutritionists, health coaches, and other health professionals have been the trusted sources of health information. Additionally, researchers have found that young adults, when they have health-related questions, typically turn to a family member who has had firsthand experience with a health condition because of their family member's close proximity and because of their past experience with, and trust in, this individual. Expertise should be a core consideration when consulting a person, website, or book for health information. The credentials and background of the person or author and conflicting interests of the author (and his or her organization) must be checked and validated to ensure the likely credibility of the health information they are conveying. While books often have implied credibility because of the peer-review process involved, self-publishing has challenged this credibility, so qualifications of book authors should also be verified. When it comes to health information, currency of the source must also be examined. When examining health information/studies presented, pay attention to the exhaustiveness of research methods utilized to offer recommendations or conclusions. Small and nondiverse sample size is often—but not always—an indication of reduced credibility. Studies that confuse correlation with causation is another potential issue to watch for. Information seekers must also pay attention to the sponsors of the research studies. For example, if a study is sponsored by manufacturers of drug Y and the study recommends that drug Y is the best treatment to manage or cure a disease, this may indicate a lack of objectivity on the part of the researchers.

The Internet is rapidly becoming one of the main sources of health information. Online forums, news agencies, personal blogs, social media sites, pharmacy sites, and celebrity "doctors" are all offering medical and health information targeted to various types of people in regard to all types of diseases and symptoms. There are professional journalists, citizen journalists, hoaxers, and people paid to write fake health news on various sites that may appear to have a legitimate domain name and may even have authors who claim to have professional credentials, such as an MD. All these sites *may* offer useful information or information that appears to be useful and relevant; however, much of the information may be debatable and may fall into gray areas that require readers to discern credibility, reliability, and biases.

While broad recognition and acceptance of certain media, institutions, and people often serve as the most popular determining factors to assess credibility of health information among young people, keep in mind that there are legitimate Internet sites, databases, and books that publish health information and serve as sources of health information for doctors, other health sites, and members of the public. For example, MedlinePlus (https://medlineplus.gov) has trusted sources on over 975 diseases and conditions and presents the information in easy-to-understand language.

The chart here presents factors to consider when assessing credibility of health information. However, keep in mind that these factors function only as a guide and require continuous updating to keep abreast with the changes in the landscape of health information, information sources, and technologies.

The chart can serve as a guide; however, approaching a librarian about how one can go about assessing the credibility of both print and online

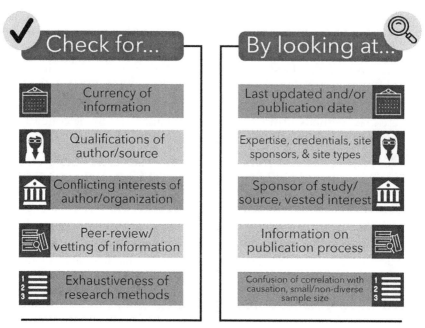

All images from flaticon.com

health information is far more effective than using generic checklist-type tools. While librarians are not health experts, they can apply and teach patrons strategies to determine the credibility of health information.

With the prevalence of fake sites and fake resources that appear to be legitimate, it is important to use the following health information assessment tips to verify health information that one has obtained (St. Jean et al., 2015, p. 151):

- **Don't assume you are right**: Even when you feel very sure about an answer, keep in mind that the answer may not be correct, and it is important to conduct (further) searches to validate the information.
- **Don't assume you are wrong**: You may actually have correct information, even if the information you encounter does not match—that is, you may be right and the resources that you have found may contain false information.
- **Take an open approach**: Maintain a critical stance by not including your preexisting beliefs as keywords (or letting them influence your choice of keywords) in a search, as this may influence what it is possible to find out.

- **Verify, verify, and verify**: Information found, especially on the Internet, needs to be validated, no matter how the information appears on the site (i.e., regardless of the appearance of the site or the quantity of information that is included).

Health literacy comes with experience navigating health information. Professional sources of health information, such as doctors, health care providers, and health databases, are still the best, but one also has the power to search for health information and then verify it by consulting with these trusted sources and by using the health information assessment tips and guide shared previously.

Mega Subramaniam, PhD
Associate Professor, College of Information
Studies, University of Maryland

REFERENCES AND FURTHER READING

American Association of School Librarians (AASL). (2009). *Standards for the 21st-century learner in action.* Chicago, IL: American Association of School Librarians.

Hilligoss, B., & Rieh, S.-Y. (2008). Developing a unifying framework of credibility assessment: Construct, heuristics, and interaction in context. *Information Processing & Management, 44*(4), 1467–1484.

Kuhlthau, C.C. (1988). Developing a model of the library search process: Cognitive and affective aspects. *Reference Quarterly, 28*(2), 232–242.

National Network of Libraries of Medicine (NNLM). (2013). Health literacy. Bethesda, MD: National Network of Libraries of Medicine. Retrieved from nnlm.gov/outreach/consumer/hlthlit.html

Ratzan, S.C., & Parker, R.M. (2000). Introduction. In C.R. Selden, M. Zorn, S.C. Ratzan, & R.M. Parker (Eds.), *National Library of Medicine current bibliographies in medicine: Health literacy.* NLM Pub. No. CBM 2000-1. Bethesda, MD: National Institutes of Health, U.S. Department of Health and Human Services.

St. Jean, B., Subramaniam, M., Taylor, N.G., Follman, R., Kodama, C., & Casciotti, D. (2015). The influence of positive hypothesis testing on youths' online health-related information seeking. *New Library World, 116*(3/4), 136–154.

St. Jean, B., Taylor, N.G., Kodama, C., & Subramaniam, M. (February 2017). Assessing the health information source perceptions of tweens using card-sorting exercises. *Journal of Information Science, 44*(2): 148–164.

Retrieved from http://journals.sagepub.com/doi/abs/10.1177/016555151 6687728 Subramaniam, M., St. Jean, B., Taylor, N.G., Kodama, C., Follman, R., & Casciotti, D. (2015). Bit by bit: Using design-based research to improve the health literacy of adolescents. *JMIR Research Protocols*, 4(2), paper e62. Retrieved from http://www.ncbi.nlm.nih.gov/pmc/articles/PMC4464334/

Valenza, J. (2016, November 26). Truth, truthiness, and triangulation: A news literacy toolkit for a "post-truth" world [Web log]. Retrieved from http://blogs.slj.com/neverendingsearch/2016/11/26/truth-truthiness-triangulation-and-the-librarian-way-a-news-literacy-toolkit-for-a-post-truth-world/

Common Misconceptions about Birth Control

1. USING CONTRACEPTION DECREASES ONE'S CHANCES OF GETTING PREGNANT IN THE FUTURE

Contraception's, or birth control's, impact on future fertility depends on the method an individual uses. For example, barrier methods like condoms or a diaphragm are devices that have no impact on a woman's menstrual cycle or a man's ability to produce sperm. Conversely, hormonal methods, including short-acting varieties (e.g., oral contraceptive pills [OCPs], the patch, or the vaginal ring) and long-acting, reversible methods (e.g., the injection of depo-medroxyprogesterone or the contraceptive implant), directly impact a woman's natural secretion of hormones and, consequently, ovulation, the character of her cervical mucus or the thickness of her uterine lining. In contrast, hormonal methods like the intrauterine device can contain hormones that work locally or directly on the uterine lining, and their hormones are not systemically absorbed, thereby not impacting fertility or ovulation. Therefore, depending on the type of contraception used, it may take several weeks or months for a woman to return to her normal ovulation or menstrual pattern after stopping any of the various hormonal methods. Sterilization, however, is intended to remove the potential of pregnancy occurring, permanently eliminating a man's or woman's fertility. In addition to reading the "Return to Fertility" section of many of the methods covered in this book, see Question 10 for more information.

2. I DON'T NEED BIRTH CONTROL BECAUSE I HAVE SEX ONLY DURING MY "SAFE" NON-FERTILE TIME OF THE MONTH

Some women have menstrual cycles that are regular and predictable each month. In addition, some women have obvious, repetitive physiologic signs or symptoms (e.g., changes in the cervical mucus, breast tenderness) that reliably alert them when ovulation is occurring or when they are most fertile. However, a woman's menstrual cycle can be altered by various factors including stress, illness, medication, weight loss or gain, or exercise. Because the menstrual cycle can vary, a woman can become pregnant unintentionally during times she thought were "safe." Any time a woman engages in unprotected sex, she is at risk for pregnancy or possibly contracting a sexually transmitted disease (STD). Women who want to avoid the possibility of pregnancy (or STDs), even those women who believe they have a predictable safe time during their menstrual cycle, should use a barrier method like condoms to provide an additional layer of protection against pregnancy occurring. For more information, see Questions 1–5, 12, and 23–25.

3. YOUR BODY NEEDS A BREAK FROM BIRTH CONTROL PILLS OCCASIONALLY

Birth control pills, or OCPs, are taken daily to provide a consistent level of hormones, or a predictable, controlled fluctuation of hormones, in a woman's bloodstream. Formulations of OCPs have evolved over the past two decades, and today's varieties contain safe doses of hormones to effectively prevent pregnancy and avoid unnecessary, and harmful, side effects. Because the available formulations are safer and able to provide doses of hormones that are ideal for an individual woman, there is no need for breaks; women can use OCPs indefinitely if they are free of any negative side effects. Women may take a break from OCP use, however, to become pregnant but can easily resume using OCPs later. See Questions 31–37 for more information about OCPs.

4. PREGNANCY CAN HAPPEN ONLY IF BOTH PARTNERS HAVE AN ORGASM

Fertilization occurs when a male sperm unites with a female egg. The intricate balance of hormones in a woman's body regulates ovulation, or the release of an egg, monthly. Therefore, a woman ovulates spontaneously, typically one time each month. A male creates sperm in his testes. However, that sperm cannot reach an egg unless sexual activity happens, and a forceful ejaculation occurs to deposit semen into the vagina. Forceful ejaculation in men is possible only with a male orgasm. A male orgasm is necessary for the sperm to leave a man's body and be available to unite with an egg. A female orgasm, in contrast, is not required for fertilization to occur. See Questions 1–2 for a detailed explanation of how the menstrual cycle works and how and when pregnancy can occur.

5. DOUCHING AFTER SEX PREVENTS PREGNANCY

Douching is intended to lavage the vagina with water, other fluids, or medicated solutions for personal hygiene or select medical conditions. Douching, however, cannot reach up into the cervix, nor can it wash out sperm that have already passed through the cervix, are in the uterus, or are traveling toward or in the fallopian tubes. Douching works by using pressure to squeeze water or other liquids forcefully into the vagina; forcing fluids into the vagina can propel any sperm in the vagina toward the cervix and, consequently, allow them to enter the cervix or uterus. Douching can change the pH of the vagina, cause vaginal irritation, or promote the improper growth of various vaginal microorganisms that can lead to vaginal infections. Douching should be avoided unless prescribed by a health-care practitioner. See Questions 1–3 for more information.

QUESTIONS AND ANSWERS

The Menstrual Cycle

1. How does the menstrual cycle happen each month?

A woman's monthly period, or the predictable days of vaginal bleeding that occurs about the same time each month, is called her menstruation. This monthly bleeding is the shedding or sloughing of the lining of the uterus when conception (or pregnancy) does not occur. Most menstrual periods last three to five days. The menstrual cycle encompasses all the different hormonal and physical changes a woman's body goes through from the first day of one month's menstrual bleeding (i.e., the first day of bleeding) to the first day of the next month's menstrual bleeding. However, the menstrual cycle is more than just the actual menstrual period; it is an intricate balance of hormones that work together in a cyclical fashion to promote ovulation, fertilization, or potential pregnancy.

Most women can accurately count the days from the beginning of one period to the beginning of the next. Typical menstrual cycles range from 21 to 35 days, with the average menstrual cycle lasting 28 days. During the menstrual cycle, important body chemicals called hormones rise and fall at different points to prepare a woman's body for pregnancy. This rise and fall of specific hormones is what regulates, or controls, the menstrual cycle.

At the beginning of the menstrual cycle, levels of the key female hormone, estrogen, begin to rise. Estrogen is produced in the ovaries, adrenal glands, and fat tissue. The rise of a stimulating hormone called luteinizing hormone causes estrogen to be produced in those specific areas, thereby increasing the level of estrogen in the bloodstream. As estrogen levels rise, the lining of the uterus responds and begins to grow and thicken. While the uterine lining is growing, one of a woman's ovaries begins to mature an egg, or ovum. By about day 14 or 15 of a typical 28-day menstrual cycle, the egg is released from the ovary, hence the term "ovulation." Women with varying, or unpredictable, menstrual cycles, in contrast, may ovulate before or after day 14. It is within the two to three days prior to ovulation, the day of ovulation, or one to two days immediately following ovulation that a woman is most likely to become pregnant.

After the egg leaves the ovary, it travels down the fallopian tube toward the uterus. Hormone levels continue to rise, and the thickened uterine lining is maintained. The surge of hormones changes a woman's natural cervical mucus to become thinner and more slippery to allow sperm to travel easily up into the uterus to meet the egg for fertilization. If a woman has sex during this time, and semen is ejaculated into the vagina, the sperm cells have a convenient path into the uterus to unite with the egg that was released. When the sperm and egg unite, fertilization occurs. The fertilized egg continues traveling down the fallopian tube toward the uterus. The thickened uterine lining is an ideal place for the fertilized egg to embed for nourishment as it continues to develop at a rapid pace.

If the egg is not fertilized, it will break apart on its own. The previously rising hormone levels in a woman's body abruptly drop. This rapid change in hormone levels causes the thickened uterine lining to break apart and shed. The shedding of the uterine lining is sporadic and occurs over several hours. Women will notice the shedding as the onset of their monthly menstrual period where bleeding occurs for about two to five days (i.e., a woman's "period"). This shedding of the uterine lining is day 1 of that month's menstrual period, signaling the end of one menstrual cycle and the onset of the next menstrual cycle.

2. What hormones are involved in the menstrual cycle?

The hormones that are involved in regulating, and maintaining, a woman's menstrual cycle occur because of a delicate balance between a woman's endocrine system and her female sex organs. The endocrine system involves several glands or organs. These organs include the pituitary gland in the brain, the thyroid gland, the pancreas, and the ovaries in a female. The endocrine system is an intricate network where certain hormones trigger glands or organs to secrete other unique hormones or to stop secreting them. Known as the "feedback mechanism," specific hormones (or stimulating hormones) get secreted at key times that stimulate glands or organs to secrete their hormones. Once the levels of stimulating hormones drop, secretion of specific hormones from a gland or organ also drops. Similarly, the endocrine system is sensitive enough to detect high levels or surges of hormones and, therefore, turn off glands or organs from secreting further hormones until the delicate balance of hormones within the system returns to equilibrium.

The pituitary gland in the brain generates two hormones: follicle stimulating hormone (FSH) and luteinizing hormone (LH). FSH and LH have a direct impact on a woman's ovary. FSH stimulates the ovarian follicle, causing an egg to grow. It also triggers the production of estrogen in the follicle. The rise in estrogen tells the pituitary gland to stop producing FSH and to start making more LH. The shift to LH causes the egg to be released from the ovary, a process called ovulation. Therefore, FSH and LH work together to cause a new egg to mature and be released from the ovarian follicle each month. As the follicle matures, however, it also produces two important female sex hormones: estrogen and progesterone. Estrogen and progesterone, therefore, regulate a woman's menstrual cycle and fertility.

Estrogen

Estrogen is produced in the ovaries. The primary function of estrogens is development of female secondary sexual characteristics. These include the breasts, development of pubic hair and bone structure, the monthly development of the endometrium, and regulation of the menstrual cycle. During puberty, the ovaries begin releasing estrogen hormones with each monthly menstrual cycle. Estrogen levels rise suddenly halfway through the cycle (due to the feedback mechanism between the pituitary gland in the brain and the ovaries). The level of estrogen in a woman's body increases, and that increase causes a rapid rise in LH (the "LH surge"). This LH surge causes the dominant follicle to rupture and release the mature egg from the ovary, which triggers the release of an egg, or ovulation. Once ovulation has occurred, the ruptured follicle forms a corpus luteum that produces high levels of progesterone. The increased levels of progesterone cause estrogen levels to quickly decline. However, what estrogen is left continues to prepare the uterus for pregnancy. If the egg is not fertilized, estrogen and progesterone levels continue to drop, and on day 28, the menses begin.

During the monthly menstrual cycle, estrogen produces an environment suitable for fertilization of an egg by a sperm cell, implantation in the uterine lining, and nourishment of an early embryo. Estrogen is the hormone responsible for the growth and development of a woman's secondary sex characteristics (e.g., breast development, the growth of armpit and pubic hair, and the regulation of a woman's menstrual cycle and reproductive system). However, there are different kinds of estrogen, and each plays a unique role in a woman's reproductive cycle. The types of estrogen include the following:

Estrone (E1)—a weak form of estrogen and the only type found in women after menopause. Small amounts of estrones are present in most tissues of the body, but most are found in fat and muscle tissues. A woman's body can convert estrone into estradiol (E2) and, conversely, estradiol into estrone.

Estradiol (E2)—the strongest type of estrogen. Estradiol is a steroid hormone (i.e., a hormone produced in the testes, ovaries, or adrenal cortex from cholesterol and travels to target cells in other parts of the body). Steroid hormones cause a variety of changes in the areas they target. Estrogen as a steroid hormone, for example, targets breast tissue and causes growth and development of the breasts.

Estriol (E3)—the weakest of the estrogens. It is a waste product made after a woman's body uses estradiol. Significant amounts of estriol are made only during pregnancy. Estriol cannot be converted to estradiol or estriol.

Estrogen, then, exerts an effect on a woman's reproductive organs:

Ovaries—estrogen helps stimulate the growth of an egg within the ovarian follicle each month.

Uterus—estrogen enhances and maintains the mucus membrane that lines the uterus. Estrogen increases the size of the endometrium (the inner lining of the uterus) along with enhancing blood flow, protein content, and enzymatic activity within the uterus. Estrogen also stimulates the muscles in the uterus to develop and contract, specifically the contractions of the uterine muscles that help rid the uterus of dead tissue (i.e., the thickened endometrium that was not needed for implantation) during menstruation (the monthly menstrual period or menstrual bleeding).

Fallopian tubes—estrogen is responsible for the growth of a thick, muscular wall inside the fallopian tubes. This muscle wall contracts and transports an egg to ultimately unite with a sperm cell.

Cervix—estrogen regulates the flow and thickness (or viscosity) of the uterine mucus. The mucus from the cervix enhances the movement of a sperm cell to an egg to enable fertilization.

Vagina—estrogen thickens the vaginal walls and increases the acidity of the vagina. The increased vaginal acidity reduces bacterial growth and, ultimately, the occurrence of bacterial vaginal infections. Estrogen also helps promote the vaginal tissues to secrete a natural lubricant to enhance, and facilitate, sexual activity.

Breasts—estrogen, in conjunction with other hormones, is responsible for the growth of the breasts during adolescence. Estrogen also plays an important role in lactation and in stopping the production and flow of breast milk when breastfeeding ceases.

Progesterone

Progesterone, like estrogen, is also a steroid hormone. It is produced by the corpus luteum in the ovary, which is a temporary endocrine gland that a woman's body produces after ovulation during the second half of the menstrual cycle. Progesterone's role is to prepare the endometrium for a potential pregnancy after ovulation; it triggers the endometrium to thicken and be able to receive and nourish a fertilized egg. Conversely, it also prohibits contractions of the uterine muscle that would reject, or expel, an egg. As the levels of progesterone rise due to the corpus luteum, ovulation ceases. Only one egg, typically, is released each month at one time.

If pregnancy does not occur, the corpus luteum begins to break down, and progesterone levels drop. The sudden change in progesterone causes menstruation to occur. However, if conception occurs, progesterone continues to stimulate a woman's body to develop the blood vessels in the endometrium that will develop the placenta and ultimately nourish a growing fetus. The high levels of progesterone during pregnancy cause a woman's body to stop maturing or releasing eggs from the ovarian follicle and helps prepare the breasts for milk production.

There are several types of progestins, or forms of progesterone. The progestins can also be synthetically derived or created in a controlled environment by drug companies. Most synthetic derivatives of progesterone are derivatives of the male hormone testosterone (known as 19-nortestosterone derivatives). Those 19-nortestosterone derivatives can be further divided into two families: estranes and gonanes.

Estrane family—first-generation progesterone that consists of norethindrone and other progestins that metabolize into, or become, norethindrone.

Gonane family—includes second-generation progesterones that have varying degrees of androgenic (i.e., male hormones that are able to be converted into female hormones in a woman's body) and estrogenic activities. These include common progesterones like levonorgestrel and norgestrel. Newer gonanes, or third-generation progestins (e.g., desogestrel and norgestimate), have the least androgenic effects. A fourth-generation progestin, drospirenone, differs from other progesterones because it is a derivative of 17a-spironolactone. The third- and fourth-generation progesterones (i.e., norgestimate, desogestrel, and drospirenone) are highly selective and possess minimal androgenic properties (e.g., irregular periods, acne, oily skin, thinning hair, thickened body hair, or weight gain).

3. Why is it so important to follow my menstrual cycle in relation to my choice of birth control?

The menstrual cycle occurs in three phases: follicular, ovulatory, and luteal. The follicular phase starts on the first day of menstruation and ends with ovulation. Prompted by the hypothalamus, the pituitary gland releases follicle stimulating hormone (FSH). This hormone stimulates the ovary to produce around 5–20 follicles (tiny nodules or cysts), which bead on the surface. Each follicle houses an immature egg. Usually, only one follicle will mature into an egg, while the others die. This can occur around day 10 of a 28-day cycle. The growth of the follicles stimulates the lining of the uterus to thicken in preparation for possible pregnancy.

The ovulatory phase is the release of a mature egg from the surface of the ovary. This usually occurs mid-cycle, around two weeks or so before menstruation starts. During the follicular phase, the developing follicle causes a rise in the level of estrogen. The hypothalamus in the brain recognizes these rising levels and releases a chemical called gonadotropin-releasing hormone. This hormone prompts the pituitary gland to produce high levels of luteinizing hormone (LH) and FSH. Within two days, ovulation is triggered by the high levels of LH. The egg is steered into the fallopian tube and toward the uterus by waves of small, hair-like projections. The life span of the typical egg is only around 24 hours. Unless it meets a sperm during this time, it will die.

During ovulation, the egg bursts from its follicle, but the ruptured follicle stays on the surface of the ovary. For the next two weeks or so, the follicle transforms into a structure known as the corpus luteum, hence the beginning of the luteal phase. This structure starts releasing progesterone, along with small amounts of estrogen. This combination of hormones maintains the thickened lining of the uterus, waiting for a fertilized egg to implant. If a fertilized egg implants in the lining of the uterus, it produces the hormones that are necessary to maintain the corpus luteum. This includes human chorionic gonadotrophin, the hormone that is detected in a urine test for pregnancy. The corpus luteum keeps producing the raised levels of progesterone that are needed to maintain the thickened lining of the uterus. If pregnancy does not occur, the corpus luteum withers and dies, usually around day 22 in a 28-day cycle. This drop in progesterone levels causes the lining of the uterus to fall away. This is known as menstruation. The cycle then repeats.

The menstrual cycle is an obvious signal of peak times during a month when a woman is most fertile and, therefore, likely to become pregnant. Conversely, it also signals the time when she is least likely to get pregnant if unprotected sexual intercourse occurs. Each woman who learns the nuances of her own individual menstrual cycle assists health-care practitioners with determining when to initiate or stop contraception or to recommend a form of contraception that is best suited to a woman. A variety of birth control choices exist; some are used at specific times during the menstrual cycle, while others are used throughout the duration of one menstrual cycle and into the next.

The nuances of the menstrual cycle become keenly important, for example, for women practicing the rhythm method, or natural family planning. Women practicing the rhythm method need to be acutely aware of the menstrual cycle and the various signs or symptoms their bodies relay to them about their specific times of fertility. Since the possibility of pregnancy is at its highest two to three days prior to, or the day of, ovulation, women following the rhythm method who do not want to become pregnant would avoid all sexual activity during those fertile days. Barrier methods such as the male or female condom or the diaphragm, however, could be used during these peak fertile times to prevent pregnancy. In addition, barrier methods are versatile and can be used at any time during the menstrual cycle to prevent pregnancy. Condoms not only help prevent pregnancy but also protect against transmission of sexually transmitted diseases (STDs) between partners.

Women opting for specific formulations of oral contraceptive pills (OCPs) will want to monitor for the arrival of their period each month. First, the monthly period is a reliable indicator that a woman did not become pregnant in the prior month. Second, most monthly birth control regimens end, and the next month's regimen begins, with the beginning or end of a monthly period. Some formulations or regimens of OCPs, however, allow women to skip having a monthly period or to have a menstrual period only a few times per year. Women on those specific regimens may continue to ovulate but rely on other physical signs (e.g., changes in cervical mucus, breast tenderness, abdominal discomfort, mood changes) to determine if, and when, ovulation is occurring.

Women with a predictable monthly period know when to expect vaginal bleeding and what amount of vaginal bleeding, for them, is normal. Many women falsely believe that they have a predictable, reliable "safe" time during their monthly menstrual cycle where they can have unprotected sex without worrying about the possibility of pregnancy. However, a woman's menstrual cycle can be altered by various factors, including stress, illness, medication, weight loss or gain, or exercise. Because the menstrual cycle can vary, a woman can become pregnant unintentionally during times she thought were safe. Any time a woman engages in unprotected sex, she is at risk for pregnancy or possibly contracting a STD. Women who want to avoid the possibility of pregnancy (or STDs), even those women who believe they have a predictable safe time during their menstrual cycle, should use a barrier method like condoms to provide an additional layer of protection against pregnancy occurring. In addition, the use of hormonal contraceptives can cause irregular bleeding or spotting. While most instances of irregular bleeding or spotting are normal, knowing where in the menstrual cycle they are occurring (e.g., day 10, day 14) will assist health-care practitioners to not only determine a probable cause but also design a plan for management. Changing hormonal contraceptive brands, regimens, or dosages is often done on specific days of the menstrual cycle.

Women using any form of contraception share a goal of preventing pregnancy from occurring. Careful attention by each woman to her menstrual cycle, including the physical or emotional changes her body goes through and on what day of her menstrual cycle they occur, assists health-care practitioners to evaluate the efficacy of prescribed contraceptive regimens or methods. Knowing, or mapping, a woman's menstrual cycle also assists health-care practitioners to quickly evaluate and diagnose pregnancy.

4. My periods are so irregular. Can I still get pregnant?

Every woman is different, including her periods. Some periods happen regularly, while others are unpredictable. On average, a woman gets her period every 24–38 days. A period usually lasts about two to eight days. Determining if a period is irregular can be difficult because the average menstrual cycle lasts about 28 days. Day 1 of a menstrual cycle is the first day of menstrual bleeding, and the last day is the day before the next period begins. Ovulation happens about two weeks before the next expected period. Therefore, if a woman experiences the average 28-day menstrual cycle, she will ovulate predictably around day 14. Many women, however, experience irregular menstrual cycles. Menstrual bleeding is considered irregular if it occurs more frequently than every 21 days or lasts longer than 8 days. Spotting, missed periods, and early or late periods are also considered irregular. Women, therefore, may have irregular periods if

- the time between each period starts to change;
- they lose more, or less, blood during a period than usual;
- the number of days that their period lasts varies greatly.

There are multiple causes for irregular periods. Common causes of irregular periods include the following:

- Having an intrauterine device
- Changing birth control pills or using certain medications
- Too much exercise
- Polycystic ovary syndrome (PCOS)
- Pregnancy or breastfeeding
- Stress
- Overactive thyroid (hyperthyroidism) or underactive thyroid (hypothyroidism)
- Thickening of or polyps on the uterine lining
- Uterine fibroids

The impact of stress or emotional factors play a significant role in menstrual regularity. Women who report high levels of stress, sadness, or depression subsequently have higher rates of menstrual irregularity. However, other subtle factors can impact menstrual irregularity. For example, eating disorders such as anorexia or bulimia, or, conversely, excessive weight gain or obesity, often make periods become irregular or disappear. Athletes, or women who overexercise, often stop menstruating as the body works to conserve energy and transforms body fat into lean muscle. Irregular periods can also be caused by diseases or conditions of the pelvic organs, such as sexually transmitted diseases. In addition, thyroid disease can cause inappropriate secretion of the hormones that trigger surges of estrogen at varying times of the month, leading to irregular bleeding or spotting throughout the menstrual cycle. Finally, the use of all forms of short- and long-acting hormonal contraception (e.g., OCPs, the vaginal ring, the patch, the contraceptive implant, the long-acting contraceptive injection) can cause various menstrual irregularities, especially when specific regimens or formulations are initiated, missed, or changed.

Many women will experience menstrual irregularity occasionally. If the issues persist, regardless of what hormonal contraceptives are in use, an evaluation by a health-care practitioner is warranted. Specifically, women who desire pregnancy, yet have a consistent pattern of irregular periods, require a comprehensive examination and evaluation by a health-care practitioner to determine if, indeed, the issues are related to infertility.

Most women, however, will not need treatment for irregular periods unless they become too troublesome or the irregularity of the menstrual cycle is too problematic for a woman who is trying to become pregnant. Certain conditions like PCOS and hypothyroidism, two common causes of irregular periods in women, can be corrected by medication, diet, and lifestyle modifications that restore the balance of hormones in the body. Classic treatment for PCOS, for example, is to use birth control pills (e.g., OCPs) or other hormones to trigger a period. Conversely, thyroid disease is often treated by replacing the missing thyroid hormone with a synthetic derivative.

A woman's chances of becoming pregnant depend on her pattern of ovulation since ovulation is the time when she is most fertile and has the highest chance of getting pregnant. A woman with irregular periods may still ovulate, just not on a regular, predictable schedule. Therefore, all women (or girls) with irregular periods can ovulate at different points from cycle to cycle. That makes it impossible for a woman to know when she is most fertile. Irregular periods also can make it hard for a woman to know if she is pregnant, since she does not know when to expect her period.

Despite irregular period, women may still ovulate and potentially become pregnant. It is possible for a woman to ovulate monthly but not have a monthly period and, therefore, become pregnant. Women who do not have regular periods are also at risk to become pregnant because ovulation is unpredictable and could start at any point during a menstrual cycle. Conversely, women can have a period without ovulation having occurred. The various forms of birth control, however, are a viable option for women with irregular periods who want to prevent pregnancy.

5. My periods are light and barely last a day. Can I still get pregnant?

A typical menstrual period begins about 12–16 days after ovulation. A woman will usually have menstrual flow, or bleeding, for about three to five days. Within those days, a woman will lose about 10 –35 mL of blood, or the equivalent of about two tablespoons, in a whole period. According to current research, the most common amount of menstrual flow measured in a laboratory from collected tampons and pads was about two tablespoons (30 mL) in a whole period. However, the amount of flow was highly variable; it ranged from a spot to over two cups (540 mL) in one period. Women who are taller, have had children, and are in perimenopause were found to have the heaviest menstrual flow during periods. The usual length of menstrual bleeding is four to six days. To better understand normal menstrual blood flow, if a woman is using common commercial, feminine sanitary products, each *soaked* normal-sized tampon or pad holds a teaspoon (5 mL) of blood. That means it is normal to soak one to seven normal-sized pads or tampons in a whole period.

Menstrual bleeding does not occur all at once. The uterine lining sloughs or sheds in small pieces over the three to five days of menstrual bleeding. A woman's menstrual bleeding may be light at times and heavier at others during the same period. The menstrual flow is highly variable and can be different each month. Women using hormonal contraceptives, such as an intrauterine device or oral contraceptive pills, and thin, underweight, or athletic women will typically have little to no bleeding or menstrual flow. Women with lighter or absent menstrual bleeding typically experience periods of shorter duration.

While lighter or shorter periods may seem ideal for women, a light or scanty period could signal issues related to infertility and impair a woman's ability to become pregnant. During the typical hormonal surges monthly, the uterine lining may respond poorly to the triggers or signals from the hormones and fail to grow and thicken properly. If an egg becomes fertilized, it needs the thickened uterine lining (or endometrium) to implant into for nourishment and growth. While there is a possibility that a woman with regular light periods could conceive spontaneously and be pregnant, often a uterine lining that is too thin will hinder implantation from occurring, and the fertilized egg will break apart. When the uterine lining is thin, there is less of it to shed and slough, causing a woman to have a light, infrequent menstrual flow each month and often a menstrual period that lasts for possibly one to three days.

Irregular periods are not always a sign of infertility. Irregular or abnormal ovulation accounts for 30–40 percent of all cases of infertility. If a woman desires pregnancy and experiences light, short periods, she should have an evaluation from a health-care practitioner. A health-care practitioner will take a thorough medical, surgical, and menstrual history from a woman to make assessments regarding her fertility or ability to conceive (i.e., become pregnant). Laboratory tests may be ordered to evaluate the levels of specific hormones in the blood at various times within the menstrual cycle. Diagnostic imaging, for example, a sonogram, may be ordered to visualize and evaluate the thickness of the uterine lining or the status of the ovaries during a menstrual cycle. This information assists a health-care practitioner to design a plan for addressing fertility issues or determine if additional testing or referral to specialists is required.

If a woman is ovulating, but irregularly, she will need to make a special effort to detecting her most fertile time. There are many ways to predict ovulation; she may need to use more than one to help figure out which is the best time for her to have sex to increase her chances of becoming pregnant. An ovulation predictor test may help her to predict the best times to have sex to increase her chances of becoming pregnant. These ovulation predictor tests work like a common pregnancy test: a woman urinates on a test strip or stick to determine when she is most fertile. However, in some women, the tests give multiple "false positives." This is especially common in women with PCOS. Another possible pitfall of using these tests when a woman has irregular cycles is that she will likely need to use more than the average number of test strips. Women with irregular periods will use the predictor tests only at specific times during their cycle when they think they may be ovulating and, therefore, use multiple test strips before they get a definitive, or presumptive, answer about their ovulatory status. Women with irregular cycles may have an ovulatory window that is longer than the average woman.

Women may consider charting their basal body temperature (BBT). BBT charting can show a woman when she ovulated. A woman can also share her BBT charts with her health-care practitioner, who may be able to use this information to make a diagnosis. Conversely, a woman may decide to forgo trying to detect ovulation and just have sex frequently throughout her menstrual cycle. There are many benefits to taking this approach. First, women with irregular periods who opt to increase the frequency of their sexual activity avoid the stress of trying to time or plan pregnancy. Predicting sexual activity around peak times of ovulation can be cumbersome for some couples. Couples would then have sex freely, and regularly, during a month and anticipate fertilization occurring from their natural sexual routine. Second, with regular, frequent sexual activity, a couple does not have to worry about missing ovulation. For example, a couple having sex three to four times a week will probably have sex on a fertile day.

If a woman is not ovulating, fertility drugs may be a viable option to improve her chances of becoming pregnant by boosting her ovulation. Even if a woman is ovulating, or ovulating irregularly or very late in her cycle, fertility treatments may help. Clomid is the most commonly prescribed drug for ovulatory dysfunction, and it has a good success rate. Another possible option is the drug letrozole. This cancer drug is used off-label to trigger ovulation. Research has found it to be possibly more effective than Clomid in women with PCOS. While not a fertility drug, another medication your doctor may suggest trying is the diabetes drug metformin. Metformin may help women with insulin resistance and PCOS ovulate on their own. If these medications do not work, a woman's health-care practitioner may suggest moving onto injectable fertility drugs (gonadotropins), intrauterine insemination treatment, or even in vitro fertilization (IVF).

If a woman's irregular cycles are caused by primary ovarian insufficiency (POI), her fertility treatment options may be limited. In many cases with POI, IVF with an egg donor is needed to conceive. This is not always the case, however. A woman should speak to her health-care practitioner about her options. If the cause for a woman's irregular cycles is a thyroid imbalance or hyperprolactinemia, treating these problems may regulate her periods and return her fertility to normal.

Fertility drugs are not a woman's only option. She may be able to make lifestyle changes, depending on the cause of her irregular cycles. For example, if she is overweight, losing some of the weight may be enough to jump-start her ovulation and help her to conceive. She may not have to lose *all* the weight; research has shown that obese women who lose just 10 percent of their weight can start ovulating on their own again. It is important to remember that some weight problems are caused by an underlying hormonal imbalance. A woman should not assume her obesity is simply attributed to improper diet or lack of physical activity. Conversely, underweight women can also experience the same effects of irregular periods. For those underweight women, gaining some weight may help regulate their cycles.

Women who overexercise are at risk for irregular periods and difficulty becoming pregnant. For those women, cutting back on their exercise routine may regulate their cycles. If a woman is an athlete, she should speak to her health-care practitioner about her options; she may need to take a break from her sport or exercise regimen to jump-start her cycles again.

Birth Control Basics

6. How long has birth control been around?

Birth control, also known as contraception and fertility control or sometimes referred to as family planning, has been in existence in various forms for millennia. Primarily plants and herbs were used both in early times and in the modern era as pharmaceuticals because of their inherent medicinal, and often contraceptive, properties. For example, evidence from as far back as 1550 BCE demonstrated that honey or acacia leaves were placed in the vagina to block semen. Hippocrates in ancient Greece wrote about plants such as willow, pomegranate, *Artemisia*, or myrrh that possess numerous contraceptive properties. In addition, in ancient China, writing from scholars documented teachings for men to learn not to ejaculate semen into the vagina.

The idea of "blocking" the vagina to prevent semen from entering began to flourish in places like the Middle East and Asia. Women were taught to insert things like lemon halves, chalk, or packed mud to block semen from reaching the womb (i.e., the uterus). Similarly, men would use animal intestine, linen sheaths, or thin layers of cured animal hide to cover the penis prior to sexual activity. These methods are most likely the first forms of the barrier contraceptive methods such as the diaphragm or condom.

In the 17th and 18th centuries sexual activity became a political, cultural, economic, and religious issue. As large numbers of the populations began to decrease due to war, disease, or famine, the need to procreate and repopulate areas or regions became apparent. However, during times when feeding, housing, and supporting families were difficult, people were eager for ways to have sexual intercourse without the risk of pregnancy. For example, in the Victorian era, women began learning natural family planning methods and timed intercourse around their menstrual periods to avoid pregnancy. Women began using a vaginal "cap" that was made of vulcanized rubber inserted into the vagina prior to sexual intercourse to prevent pregnancy.

In the United States, contraception began to be regulated around the 1870s when the Comstock Act, and the various individual state Comstock laws, passed that outlawed the distribution of information about contraception or the use of contraceptives. However, Margaret Sanger championed the cause for birth control and opened a controversial birth control clinic in 1916. Sanger would later be arrested and put on trial for distributing contraceptives. The publicity surrounding Sanger's arrest and trial ignited a birth control movement; funding from numerous donors allowed Sanger to continue her work and advocacy for birth control. Sanger would continue to face numerous legal battles, but her persistence paid off when the Comstock laws were repealed in 1938. Sanger continued to advocate for birth control, including becoming an underwriter and fund-raiser for research to create the first human birth control pill. In 1960, the first oral contraceptive, Enovid, was approved by the U.S. Food and Drug Administration (FDA).

Other forms of birth control would be developed. The intrauterine device (IUD) was first approved by the FDA in 1968, and different formulations of the oral contraceptive pill (or "the Pill") began to appear on the market. In the 1980s, the copper IUD was introduced along with the Yuzpe regimen for emergency contraception. The 1990s saw the first implantable form of contraception (Norplant), the first injectable form of contraception (Depo-Provera), the first commercially packaged emergency contraception (Plan B), and the first female condom introduced. Since 2000, the hormonal contraceptive patch (Ortho Evra), the vaginal contraceptive ring (NuvaRing), and the first transcervical female sterilization (Essure) have been developed. Evolution in birth control continues; innovations for the future include research on female-controlled methods of contraception that prevent not only pregnancy but also sexually transmitted diseases and the development of hormonal birth control methods for men.

7. What are the different kinds of birth control?

There are a variety of birth control options available for men and women. The choice of birth control depends on several factors, including medical history, any past experiences with different forms of contraception, one's lifestyle, smoking habits, menstrual cycle, current medications, plans for pregnancy in the future, one's emotional or mental health and personal choice. There is not one ideal or perfect form of birth control. A method that best works today may not be suitable for use in the future. A health-care practitioner can discuss and explain the various birth control options in detail and help determine the best method for contraception. The options for birth control can be understood best by explaining them in broad categories: natural methods, barrier methods, hormonal preparations, and permanent forms.

Natural methods refer to the practices that do not involve any medication, commercial products, or medical procedures. Most natural methods can be complex but may be possible to learn, and use, without requiring a consultation with a health-care practitioner. Natural methods include abstinence, the rhythm method, and the "pull out" technique. Abstinence is the most effective at preventing pregnancy: sexual intercourse is avoided; therefore, no chance of semen entering, or coming in contact with, the vagina exists. Other forms of intimacy are encouraged, such as kissing, hugging, or touching, but any contact or penetration between the penis and a woman's vagina or rectum is avoided. In contrast, the rhythm method allows sexual activity to happen but not on the specific days preceding, or the day of, ovulation. "Rhythm," as the method is commonly referred to, relies on a woman's accurate tracking of her menstrual cycle and acceptance or understanding that pregnancy is a possibility if her menstrual cycle is irregular or her calculations are incorrect. The withdrawal, or "pull out," method, known as *coitus interruptus,* requires the male partner to be in tune with his own body and be keenly aware when he is about to climax or orgasm (and ejaculate). When withdrawal is used during sexual activity, a man immediately ends sex by withdrawing or "pulling out" of a woman's vagina prior to reaching climax or orgasm and ejaculates his semen outside of her body. Risk for pregnancy with withdrawal is high since sperm lives in seminal fluid (i.e., "pre-cum") that is secreted immediately before and during sexual activity. In addition, ejaculated semen splashed on or near a woman's vagina could still permit sperm to enter the vagina and cause pregnancy to occur.

Given the complexity or uncertainties associated with the natural methods, many people use barrier methods. Condoms are the most popular form of barrier methods. Condoms are single use and durable for sustained events of sexual activity. When used properly and consistently, condoms are 98 percent effective at preventing pregnancy and sexually transmitted diseases. Male condoms are the most commonly used form of contraception. They are inexpensive, effective, easy to use, and available in multiple places for purchase or sometimes dispensed free in certain areas. Female condoms are also available, although not as popular as the male condom. Women, however, have been using the diaphragm for decades. The diaphragm is typically a latex cap that a woman inserts into her vagina. The diaphragm covers the cervix and prevents sperm from entering the uterus. The diaphragm is reusable and can be left in for several days, thereby allowing for multiple episodes of sexual activity. Diaphragms, however, need to be fitted and sized properly by an experienced health-care practitioner and be rechecked periodically to ensure proper fit and that the diaphragm is still intact. For people allergic to latex that is commonly found in condoms or diaphragms, spermicidal gels, lubricants, or foams offer another barrier option. Spermicides work by being inserted directly into the vagina prior to sexual intercourse or by being used to lubricate the penis prior to its entry into the vagina. The chemicals within a spermicide are meant to slow the movement of sperm that may be ejaculated into the vagina, preventing it from reaching an egg and preventing fertilization. While spermicides work well as lubricants, their reliability to prevent pregnancy when used as the sole method of birth control is low. Many people, however, combine spermicides with another method, for example, using spermicidal lubricants on the outside of a condom or inside the cap or curve of a diaphragm.

Hormonal birth control, in contrast to natural or barrier methods, works directly on the release of the hormones that control the menstrual cycle. Some preparations, such as oral contraceptive pills (OCPs or "the Pill"), are taken daily by a woman to stop ovulation from occurring, prevent the uterine lining from growing and thickening, make the uterus unwelcoming to sperm, or thicken the cervical mucus, or as a combination of all four. OCPs require an evaluation and prescription by a health-care practitioner along with follow-up at intervals to determine their efficacy or presence of any side effects. In addition, OCPs require a woman to take a pill each day, avoid missing doses, use caution with any other medications, and get a refill monthly. To minimize some of the inconveniences associated with OCPs, long-acting, reversible hormonal contraceptives such as injectable preparations, the vaginal ring, hormonal patch, and the intrauterine device (IUD) were developed. An injectable form of contraception (e.g., Depo-Provera) has specific hormones contained within a suspension that, when injected into a muscle, breaks down slowly over time, releasing a steady, yet small, quantity of hormone. A woman typically requires another injection every three months but avoids the inconvenience of taking an oral contraceptive pill daily or the risk of missing doses. The vaginal ring is a flexible, hormone-containing ring placed inside the vagina for a week at a time. Hormones are secreted from the ring and absorbed across the tissues of the vaginal walls to prevent pregnancy. Sexual activity can continue uninhibited if the ring remains in place. The hormonal patch, in contrast, is applied to any skin surface where its hormonal agents get absorbed slowly through the skin to prevent pregnancy. The hormonal patch, like the ring, is typically changed weekly. The IUD, in contrast, is inserted directly into the uterus during an in-office procedure by a health-care practitioner. The IUD works by preventing the growth and thickening of the uterine lining monthly, thereby preventing pregnancy. The advantage of the IUD is that it is a reliable form of contraception that can remain in place for years; it is not, however, intended to be permanent.

Permanent contraception can be achieved only through sterilization procedures. Options for permanent sterilization vary from minimally invasive to surgical procedures. The Essure is a transcervical procedure where a specialized insert is placed inside each fallopian tube. Scar tissue eventually forms around the inserts, thereby blocking sperm from reaching eggs. Similarly, a woman may opt for a tubal ligation where, during a minor surgical procedure, the fallopian tubes are cut and permanently "tied," or ligated, thereby preventing eggs from reaching the uterus and sperm from ever reaching the eggs. A woman who undergoes a hysterectomy, where the uterus (and sometimes the fallopian tubes and ovaries) is removed, will have permanent sterilization since the major organ (or organs) required for pregnancy is removed. Men can also undergo permanent sterilization by having a vasectomy. During this minimally invasive procedure, a structure called the vas deferens is clamped or cut from each testicle, thereby preventing sperm from mixing with semen that is ejaculated during sexual intercourse.

8. Why are most birth control methods targeted at women?

In the birth control arena, the number of options for women outnumbers the options available to, or targeted at, men. Men essentially have four options for birth control: abstinence, withdrawal, condoms, or a vasectomy. Conversely, women have barrier methods, short- and long-acting forms of hormonal contraception, and several options for permanent sterilization. The existence of these options for women, however, is a source of social and cultural controversy.

For many years women had little control over their fertility. Women would go through repeated pregnancies and childbirth, often left alone to raise children during difficult political or economic situations. The development of the oral contraceptive pill gave women control over their own fertility for the first time. Women were empowered to determine when, or if, they would become pregnant. The oral contraceptive pill gained popularity, and different formulations were created to meet the needs of a diverse group of women who were requesting them.

Oral contraceptive pills, or other forms of hormonal contraception, are effective for women. It is easier, and more reliable with a high degree of safety, to control the release of one egg from an ovary in a woman's body, or the growth of a small-to-moderate amount of tissue that makes up the internal uterine lining, than the uncertainty of trying to limit the production or potency of millions of sperm that can be present in one male's ejaculation. While innovations for male hormonal birth control are currently being researched, the current forms of hormonal contraception work most effectively and reliably on the female reproductive system, hence the ongoing targeting of women as advances in any forms of contraception are explored.

Despite the obvious focus of birth control on women, contraception is not a woman's sole responsibility. Men and women share the responsibility of birth control. Health-care practitioners emphasize educating both partners about various birth control methods, so a couple can make the informed choices that best suit their relationship. A couple can then decide how the responsibility for contraception can be shared. Examples of men assuming shared contraceptive responsibility include men purchasing condoms and having them readily available for sexual activity, assisting their partners with refilling any prescriptions for hormonal birth control, paying the fees for any visits with health-care practitioners or co-payments for prescriptions, reminding their partners to take any daily birth control pills, and joining their partners for any follow-up visits to a health-care practitioner.

9. What conditions or situations would prevent me from using birth control?

While birth control in its various forms is a highly effective, reliable, and relatively safe option for men and women, there are certain precautions or concerns that must be evaluated prior to initiating some forms of contraception. The conditions or situations assessed, however, differ based on whether the choice involves barrier methods, short- or long-acting hormonal contraceptive methods, or permanent sterilization.

Most barrier methods such as condoms or diaphragms are made from latex, rubber, or sometimes plastic material. Latex is a common material found in balloons or gloves and can be mistaken for rubber, vinyl, or plastic. Allergies to latex are common and can cause different allergic reactions ranging from localized redness, itching, or swelling to the penis or vagina to a full systemic body reaction, including anaphylaxis. Both men and women need to review if they have an allergy to latex (e.g., any previous reactions holding or blowing up latex balloons, any reactions using latex gloves). Anaphylaxis is a sudden swelling of the airway, leading to increasing difficulty breathing and eventually a life-threatening emergency. A person allergic to latex, or suspects he or she might be allergic to latex, must avoid latex condoms or diaphragms.

The various chemicals in spermicide creams, gels, or lubricants can be irritating to the tissues within the vagina or inside the opening of the penis. Allergic reactions can occur with spermicidal preparations also, ranging from localized skin irritation to full body redness, swelling, rashes, or possible anaphylaxis. Any spermicidal preparations should be tested in small amounts on different body tissues or surfaces of the skin; if any discomfort such as burning, itching, or redness is experienced or observed, discard the current preparation and explore others.

Hormonal contraceptives, including oral contraceptive pills, the vaginal ring, hormonal, or the intrauterine device, have unique precautions that need to be evaluated prior to initiating their use. First, if a woman is pregnant or thinks she might be pregnant, she should not begin any forms of hormonal contraception. Similarly, if a woman is breastfeeding, or may have surgery in the future where the risk of blood clots is increased, her hormonal birth control options may be limited. The largest risk with hormonal contraception stems from the hormones contained within the different formulations available and the effect those hormones exert on different body tissues. Hormones, for example, exert a powerful effect on the vascular system and blood vessels, which could increase the likelihood, or accelerate the process, of blood clotting. Therefore, women with a medical history that includes having had a heart attack, stroke, high blood pressure, high cholesterol, or migraines require a thorough evaluation by a health-care practitioner prior to initiating any form of hormonal contraception. In addition, women with a medical history that includes cancer, liver or gall bladder disease, obesity, unexplained vaginal bleeding, depression, or certain prescription medications will require careful screening by a health-care practitioner to ensure the safest hormonal methods are offered. Smoking poses a unique risk for women because nicotine exerts its effect on the lining of blood vessels, further increasing the possibility of women developing blood clots. Women who are smokers should consider quitting prior to exploring any form of hormonal contraception.

Permanent sterilization techniques carry precautions also. Like other methods, a woman who is actively pregnant or is undecided about her desire to end her fertility is not a candidate for permanent sterilization. If a woman has an active pelvic infection in the uterus or fallopian tubes (e.g., pelvic inflammatory disease), or an active sexually transmitted disease (STD), the sterilizing procedure will be postponed until no evidence of infection is present. Some procedures require sedation or anesthesia, so allergies to sedatives or anesthetics require a careful evaluation by a health-care practitioner while planning for, and reevaluation immediately prior to, a permanent sterilization procedure. Men, in comparison, would be poor candidates for permanent sterilization if they, too, are uncertain about their desire to end their fertility or have an active testicular infection or an STD.

10. If I use birth control now, will it affect any pregnancies in the future when I decide I want to have kids?

The purpose of birth control is to prevent pregnancy. The different forms of birth control, however, exert different effects and are for different durations. Fertility for the future depends on whether the choice of birth control was natural methods, barrier methods, or short- or long-acting hormonal contraception.

Couples using the natural methods like rhythm, or the withdrawal technique, face the possibility of pregnancy with every sexual encounter. The natural methods have no impact on fertility because they do not interfere with ovulation, the growth of the uterine lining, or the production of sperm. Instead, these methods try to minimize the opportunity for sperm to encounter an egg. Therefore, if the natural methods are abandoned and sexual activity resumes whenever it is desired, pregnancy can occur at any time.

Like the natural methods, barrier methods work by preventing the opportunity for sperm to unite with an egg. Therefore, if a barrier method is in place with each episode of sexual activity pregnancy should be avoided. However, barrier methods, like the natural methods, do not inhibit ovulation, nor any of the other processes within the male or female reproductive system. Not using a barrier method could allow pregnancy to occur immediately with any episode of sexual activity if ovulation occurred.

Hormonal methods, in contrast to natural and barrier methods, work by introducing different doses of hormones into a woman's bloodstream to suppress her monthly ovulation, prevent the growth of the uterine lining, thicken cervical mucus, make the intrauterine environment unwelcoming to sperm, or a combination of some or all effects. Short-acting hormonal contraception, such as oral contraceptive pills (OCPs), taken every day see the quickest return to fertility once they are stopped. The menstrual cycle needs to return to its prior pattern of ovulation once the hormones of low-dose or regular dose OCPs are no longer circulating within a woman's bloodstream, a process that typically takes one to two months (or one to two menstrual cycles) for fertility to recur. However, depending on the formulation of OCPs, ovulation may occur sooner or take several months to recur. Women using the hormonal vaginal ring, or the hormonal patch, require the same time frame to return to fertility as women who use OCPs; once the ring or patch is removed and not replaced, the amount of hormone a woman is exposed to immediately diminishes or is nonexistent.

Long-acting hormonal contraception like injectable Depo-Provera or an intrauterine device (IUD) faces different challenges with fertility. Injectable, long-acting preparations are intended to be a reliable birth control method because they exert their effect slowly over time. The preparations are created with an additional medication that binds with the hormones and gets slowly broken down over time by a woman's body, releasing small amounts of controlled doses of their hormonal medication. Not taking subsequent doses of the long-acting hormonal contraceptive when due is the first step toward resuming fertility. Once stopped, it may take several weeks or months for all the residual amounts of hormonal medication to be released, utilized, and eventually removed from the body. A method like the IUD, in contrast, exerts its action directly on the uterine lining to prevent its growth and thickening. Once the IUD is removed, it may be possible for couples to conceive or become pregnant immediately. However, it may take four to six months post removal for pregnancy to occur.

Permanent sterilization is intended to block all chances of pregnancy from occurring. However, some individuals attempt reversal procedures to become fertile again. Fertility varies by the type of sterilization reversed. Following a vasectomy, it may take three to six months for enough sperm to populate each ejaculation to allow pregnancy to occur. In contrast, a successful reversal of a tubal ligation with proper healing and no complications may permit pregnancy to occur within two to three months post reversal procedure.

11. Is there birth control for men only?

While men hold equal responsibility for birth control, the options for men related to birth control are few. Men have the options of barrier methods and permanent sterilization; a hormonal option for men has yet to be made available. However, innovations related to male contraception continue to be forged, which offer promising options for the future.

There are millions of sperm contained within a man's ejaculation after one episode of sexual activity. If sex is unprotected, the likelihood for one of those millions of sperm uniting with a single female egg is high. To avoid conception or pregnancy, men need to prevent any sperm from their ejaculation (sperm is contained within the semen that is ejaculated) from reaching the uterus. The only options available for men include the withdrawal method, using the male condom, or a vasectomy. Success with each method varies; withdrawal has the lowest success rate, while condoms and permanent sterilization offer the most reliable birth control option.

Within the scientific community, advances have been made to widen the options available for male birth control. Hormonal, long-acting birth control for men is currently under investigation in the United States. Using an injectable combination of testosterone and a synthetic form of a female reproductive hormone (norethisterone enanthate), a man would receive an intramuscular injection every eight weeks, similar to a woman's injection of Depo-Provera, to stop the testicles from producing testosterone and, ultimately, sperm. Research on this form of hormonal contraception, however, has been slow and lacking funds for advancing the research. Similarly, outside the United States biomedical scientists have developed a polymer gel that can be injected into the sperm-carrying tubes attached to the testicles. This polymer, once injected, thickens, and its positive chemical charges buffer the negative chemical charge of sperm, thereby destroying the sperm's head and tail leading to infertility. This innovation potentially offers long-acting birth control for men; an additional dose of the polymer later renders the original dose inactive and allows fertility to return. Like the injectable hormonal form of male birth control, additional testing and research is needed to determine the efficacy of both innovations. However, outside of scientific scrutiny, both methods face controversy from pharmaceutical and barrier method industries due to the potential financial impact each new method could have on profits for previously established, profitable, forms of birth control.

12. Do I need to worry about sexually transmitted diseases if I'm on birth control?

Sexually transmitted diseases (STDs) are caused by the transmission of harmful microorganisms, such as bacteria, viruses, fungi, or protozoans, that cause diseases or conditions to male or female genital tract organs or structures. The different birth control methods are effective at preventing conception or pregnancy from occurring, but they do nothing to protect a person from STDs. Condoms, however, are the only form of birth control that serves a dual purpose of preventing pregnancy and minimizing the transmission of harmful microorganisms that cause STDs. Therefore, the risk for STDs exists for anyone having unprotected sexual activity. The same precautions one would take with any new sex partner need to be used if a man or woman is using any type of birth control.

Natural methods and barrier methods, except for the male and female condom, still permit seminal fluid or semen to come in contact with the tissues in and outside the vagina. A diaphragm may block sperm from entering the cervix or uterus, but a sufficient amount of semen can remain within the vagina or meet the cervix after the diaphragm is removed. Spermicides, similarly, do not form a barrier to protect the cervix or vagina; harmful microorganisms can still meet vulnerable tissues of the vagina or cervix.

Women who use hormonal contraceptive methods, however, often fail to use any form of barrier method in addition to their hormonal form of birth control. Women become focused on preventing pregnancy and neglect to consider the possibility of contracting an STD. Having unprotected sex, regardless of the type of hormonal contraception a woman may be using, exposes her to any harmful microorganisms her partner may be carrying, thereby increasing a woman's risk of contracting an STD. Hormonal methods are intended for women who are either in a mutually monogamous relationship where both partners are screened for STDs or who are willing to use hormonal methods for pregnancy prevention and a barrier method such as condoms for any sexual activity with new, random, infrequent, or multiple partners.

Permanent sterilization, like hormonal methods, offers no protection against STDs. While unprotected sex with someone who has undergone a permanent sterilization procedure makes the possibility of pregnancy remote, the possibility of transmitting an STD exists if one or both partners are carrying the harmful microorganisms that cause an STD or have an active STD already. The use of a barrier method like condoms is recommended for anyone who has undergone a sterilization procedure and is engaging in sexual activity with any new, random, infrequent, or multiple partners.

13. Does using birth control put me at a higher risk for cancer?

The risk for cancer related to contraception primarily surrounds the use of hormonal methods of birth control. The hormonal methods are typically formulated with different doses of the female hormones estrogen or progesterone. Some forms of the hormones are in their natural state, while others are synthetic formulations of estrogen, progesterone, or other hormonal combinations intended to make various forms of birth control more effective with less untoward side effects. Regardless of individual formulations, the hormones in birth control target specific tissues or organs in a woman's body: the ovaries, the uterus, and indirectly breast tissue.

The use of birth control pills has been implicated as a risk factor for the development of breast cancer. Current research supports that the risk of developing breast cancer is slightly increased in women who currently use birth control pills, or used birth control pills in the past, compared to women who never used birth control pills. Similarly, a woman's risk of cervical cancer increases during the time she is using birth control pills. Her risk of cervical cancer is at its highest if she has been on birth control for five or more years. The risk for cervical cancer quickly decreases once a woman stops using birth control pills.

In contrast to the increased risk for breast cancer or cervical cancer with birth control pills, a woman's risk for ovarian cancer is thought to be decreased if she uses birth control pills. Current research supports that birth control pills may also reduce the risk for cancers for women who carry the *BRCA-1* and *BRCA-2* gene mutations. Women without either mutation, however, continue to have an increased risk of breast cancer because of birth control pill use.

Because links to various cancers have been discovered with the use of hormonal methods of birth control, a thorough health history and evaluation by a health-care practitioner precedes initiating hormonal methods such as birth control pills. Included in this evaluation are a review of a woman's family history of cancers in her primary relatives and an assessment of her individual risk of developing cancer herself. Health-care practitioners will discuss various birth control options and alternatives for a woman. If a woman wants to use hormonal methods once being informed of the risks, benefits, and alternatives, health-care practitioners will work with the patient to select a formulation that contains the safest, lowest amounts of hormones that will be effective at preventing pregnancy.

14. Can I get birth control on my own, or do I need an examination and prescription?

Birth control has become more accessible in recent decades. Barriers or restrictions to obtaining birth control were removed by women's health advocates, who argued that more women would access birth control options if obtaining it was less cumbersome. Today, a physical examination or prescription is not always required to initiate birth control.

Men and women can freely access barrier methods like condoms or spermicides. There are a variety of commercial products available that are sold in convenient locations, including retail stores and pharmacies. The diaphragm, however, requires a woman to have a pelvic examination by a health-care practitioner to determine which size and style is most appropriate based on her body type and vaginal anatomy.

Certain forms of hormonal contraception no longer require a pelvic examination prior to initiating. However, a health-care practitioner will want to do a thorough review of a woman's medical, surgical, and menstrual histories so the most appropriate formulation of hormonal contraception can be prescribed. A pelvic examination is not needed if the woman is a teenager. A pelvic examination prior to prescribing hormonal contraception is recommended if a woman presents with abdominal pain, abnormal vaginal bleeding, or discharge or believes she might have a sexually transmitted disease (STD). All sexually active men and women should have regular STD screenings to identify and treat any STDs early; a pelvic examination may be necessary for some women to perform an appropriate screening. A prescription may be necessary for women to obtain hormonal contraception. Depending on the state a woman lives in, some offices and clinics are permitted to dispense hormonal contraception; other states require pharmacies dispense any medication, including hormonal contraception. For states where pharmacies are required to obtain hormonal contraception, prescriptions to begin and refill the medication are necessary.

Long-acting hormonal contraception requires a prescription but not always a full pelvic examination by a health-care practitioner. For example, to use an intrauterine device (IUD), a woman needs a pelvic examination and then a minor procedure in a health-care practitioner's office or clinic to insert the IUD safely. In some states, a woman has an examination first and then obtains a prescription for an IUD that she fills at a pharmacy; she brings the IUD with her to the follow-up appointment, and that is the IUD that gets inserted. Conversely, some health-care practitioners or clinics keep a supply of IUDs and can dispense, and insert, those at the point of care. Similarly, injectable, long-acting hormonal contraception, such as Depo-Provera, may require a prescription to refill the medication every three months. Women in some areas fill the prescription and bring the syringe of medication to the health-care practitioner's office or clinic for injection. In other states, health-care practitioners may dispense and administer the medication immediately at the point of care. Since other forms of hormonal contraception such as the vaginal ring or hormonal patch are self-managed by each woman, a prescription is often needed for a pharmacist to dispense the product to her and then for the subsequent refills depending on the policies of the pharmacy.

Sterilization, in contrast to all other forms of birth control, requires a thorough evaluation and discussion with a health-care practitioner. Sterilization in any form for men or women is a minor surgical procedure; examinations by a health-care practitioner are required, but prescriptions are often not applicable.

15. Is birth control covered by insurance?

With the passage of the Patient Protection and Affordable Care Act (the ACA, or commonly called "Obamacare") in 2010, birth control became more accessible and affordable for both men and women. In most states, if one has health insurance, birth control is considered a covered benefit; obtaining birth control should result in no additional expenses or co-payments. However, the terms of the ACA apply only to health insurance plans that are not considered "grandfathered"; those plans were permitted to maintain their previous levels of coverage and were not required to conform to the terms outlined in the ACA. It is best to contact one's insurance company directly and inquire if visits to a health-care practitioner, and prescriptions for birth control, are covered. In addition, pharmacists and their staff are valuable resources for determining what types or brands of birth control are covered by specific insurance plans. Some plans, for example, cover only limited birth control options or only specific brands of birth control medications or generic formulations.

For those without health insurance or the ability to attain it, Medicaid may be a viable option for men and women. Medicaid programs offered free birth control and contraceptive services from a health-care practitioner prior to the passage of the ACA and continue to do so. Medicaid programs, however, are administered and funded by each individual state; what is covered under each Medicaid program varies from state to state. Medicaid programs are not required to cover all Food and Drug Administration–approved birth control methods. It is best to contact one's state Medicaid office to find out what services or birth control options are covered.

There are important things to consider regarding the use of insurance to cover the cost of birth control. For example, certain religious organizations are exempt from requirements to provide coverage for birth control or sterilization. In addition, if one is covered under one's parents' insurance plan, it might be difficult to obtain birth control privately without a parent discovering that birth control is being used. Fortunately, organizations such as Planned Parenthood, college or other community clinics, exist that offer men and women expert care and access to birth control options at affordable prices. These organizations work with individuals to find affordable sources of health care if needed and provide support, education, privacy, and confidentiality to their patients.

16. Will my partner know if I'm on birth control?

Using birth control can be obvious or discreet. For example, the use of condoms, regardless of whether the male or female condom is used, is a very visible form of birth control, hence difficult to conceal. In contrast, forms of hormonal contraception can be used privately. The choice of birth control method determines whether a sex partner will know if a form of birth control is in use.

The barrier methods are the most obvious forms of birth control. Condoms are very conspicuous when applied to an erect penis or unrolled inside a vagina. Similarly, spermicidal creams are typically white or creamy in appearance and, therefore, can be visible at the vaginal opening or within the vagina. Clear spermicidal gels are less obvious to see.

Hormonal patches, like condoms, are easily visible because they adhere outside the body. The adhesive square or disc of medication can be easily recognized on an area of skin. The diaphragm is not visible at the vaginal opening, but it may be felt during intercourse by the tip of a penis or discovered during foreplay with oral sex or by a partner's fingers probing the vagina. The vaginal contraceptive ring, while not visible outside the vagina, may also be palpated during aggressive foreplay or discovered during oral sex. The intrauterine device, although a form of long-acting birth control, has two thin strings that deliberately hang a few inches outside the cervix. Men have reported that they can feel the strings scraping or touching the tip of their penis during sex.

Hormonal birth control that is taken in pill form orally or injected is the most discreet form of birth control. It is easy to take a daily pill or injection every three months privately without a sex partner knowing. If a man or woman has undergone permanent sterilization, there is no way a sex partner will be able to know or tell with the naked eye or during sexual activity.

What is important to stress is that the use of birth control should be discussed openly between sex partners. The use of birth control should not be the sole responsibility of one partner only. Depending on the number of sex partners each partner has had, and the frequency of intercourse both partners are having both together and with other people, it may necessitate the use of additional birth control methods such as barrier methods like condoms to prevent transmission of harmful microorganisms that can lead to sexually transmitted diseases. The use of birth control should be an open, honest discussion between sex partners.

17. If I start using birth control, what type of monitoring or follow-up do I need?

The type and timing of any follow-up or monitoring with a health-care practitioner needed following the initiation of birth control depend on the birth control method chosen. Some birth control options require no follow-up, some require only checking in with a health-care practitioner, and others may require several follow-up appointments with a health-care practitioner.

The barrier methods are the simplest forms of birth control and require no follow-up visits after initiating their use. Once instructed on the proper and consistent use of condoms and spermicides, a person using them does not need to return to see a health-care practitioner. Men and women can easily obtain condoms or spermicides in a store or pharmacy. If a woman chooses a diaphragm, however, some follow-up with a health-care practitioner is often scheduled so that proper fit, ease of insertion and removal, and satisfaction with the diaphragm overall can be assessed. If the diaphragm needs to be resized or refitted, a new prescription can be provided and filled.

Hormonal contraception, unlike the barrier methods, often requires a follow-up visit after initiating its use and then annually thereafter. The concern with hormonal contraception is its potential side effects; it is important for women to be evaluated and educated regularly about the potential dangerous side effects and their early warning signs. Follow-up visits allow for evaluation of any menstrual irregularities and an opportunity for a health-care practitioner to switch a woman to a different formulation of birth control pills or a different method.

The follow-up for any long-acting birth control methods varies based on the specific method used. For example, the hormonal patch or the vaginal ring, like oral contraceptive pills (OCPs), requires a check-in with a health-care practitioner after several weeks' use to evaluate if any unexpected or dangerous side effects or symptoms may be present. Like OCPs, a yearly gynecologic examination provides the opportunity for a health-care practitioner to evaluate the hormonal patch's or vaginal ring's effectiveness and provide a woman with a prescription to obtain additional refills of her birth control option. In contrast, injectable Depo-Provera requires some form of follow-up every three months so that a woman can receive her next injection of medication at its scheduled time. While some pharmacists can administer the injection, follow-up typically occurs in a health-care practitioner's office or clinic. In addition to providing the injection, the health-care practitioner assesses women for any warning signs of dangerous side effects related to using the medication, weight gain, and reviews blood pressure and heart rate readings prior to each reinjection as part of the ongoing monitoring.

Permanent sterilization procedures, based on the fact that they are minor surgical procedures, typically require scheduled follow-up after the procedure is completed to assess for healing of the surgical wounds. Men and women following a sterilization procedure are advised to use an additional form of contraception such as condoms until sterility is confirmed. Confirming sterility occurs three months or more following the sterilization procedure by a health-care practitioner. For men, a semen analysis will be performed to monitor for a significant decrease in, or absence of, sperm in the ejaculation. Women who have the Essure device inserted may undergo a hysterosalpingogram (a radiologic procedure that examines the fallopian tubes and uterus) to identify, and confirm, the occluded ends of the fallopian tubes exist and are not patent to allow pregnancy to occur.

18. If I've had a baby, how soon after delivery can I begin using birth control?

The decision of which birth control method to use, and when to use it, following the birth of a baby depends on a few factors. First, if a woman plans to breastfeed her baby, her choices of birth control will be narrowed because several forms of hormonal contraception can interfere with lactation. Second, a woman must decide if she wants to resume a method of birth control she used previously or wants to try a new method. Regardless of what method a woman chooses, it is important that she discuss her plans for birth control with her health-care provider prior to delivery. A period of six to eight weeks' healing will follow post-delivery where sex, and sexual activity, is discouraged. However, it is best that a woman be prepared when sexual activity resumes so that she does not immediately become pregnant again.

Barrier methods are the most popular form of birth control following delivery of a baby. Condoms, for example, are affordable, convenient, and effective at preventing pregnancy when used properly and consistently. A woman or couple can keep an ample supply of condoms on hand for resuming sexual activity. However, if a woman wants to resume using a diaphragm, she will need an examination by her health-care practitioner post-delivery to check the fit and size of the diaphragm before it is used following delivery of a baby; childbirth changes the tone and shape of the vagina, so a different type or size of diaphragm may be necessary.

If a woman is considering hormonal contraception, she will typically need to wait about four weeks following delivery. After childbirth, levels of estrogen in a woman's bloodstream are high; adding estrogen from various forms of birth control such as oral contraceptive pills (OCPs), hormonal patches, or vaginal rings could put a woman at risk for blood clots or other dangerous side effects. Estrogen levels begin to decline by approximately four weeks following delivery of a baby, so it is safer to initiate either combined hormonal OCPs, the hormonal patch, or the vaginal ring a month or more following delivery. If a woman is breastfeeding, estrogen-containing forms of birth control are avoided until breast milk production and supply is well established; estrogen may reduce the quantity and quality of breast milk. However, if a woman is breastfeeding, she may opt to use the "mini pill," or a progestin-only form of OCP. While the mini pill is a good alternative for breastfeeding women, the mini pill requires a steady dose of hormone to be present in a woman's bloodstream; the mini pill must be taken at the same time each day as prescribed, without missing a dose, or its contraceptive effect is diminished.

Long-acting hormonal contraception can be initiated at the time of delivery of a baby or immediately thereafter. For example, some practitioners will insert an intrauterine device (IUD) immediately following delivery of a baby and the placenta because there is optimal visualization of the cervix to allow accurate placement of the IUD. Most health-care practitioners will opt to insert an IUD from four to six weeks following delivery to minimize the risk of improper placement or infection. Conversely, a woman can receive her first injection of Depo-Provera, a progestin-only form of birth control, immediately after giving birth or prior to discharge from the hospital without interfering with her ability to breastfeed. In addition, Depo-Provera taken immediately after delivery provides a woman 12 weeks of consistent birth control, allowing her to explore, and initiate, other birth control options by the time of her first post-delivery, follow-up appointment with her health-care practitioner, or approximately 6 weeks after delivery.

Permanent sterilization procedures require advanced planning to be implemented. For example, a woman may be a candidate for a tubal ligation with a Cesarean section delivery. The sterilization procedure can be completed during the Cesarean section surgery. Otherwise, permanent sterilization procedures would be planned after healing from delivery of a baby has occurred. Other methods of birth control, for example, barrier methods, would be used until a permanent sterilization procedure could be completed.

19. Does breastfeeding work to prevent pregnancy?

Women who breastfeed their newborn will often experience a delay in their return to fertility. Known as "lactational amenorrhea," breastfeeding contributes to preventing pregnancy because the baby feeding regularly at the breast keeps levels of the hormone prolactin high which, in turn, promotes lactation or the continued production of breast milk. Increased prolactin suppresses ovulation. Therefore, normal estrogen levels are decreased.

When ovulation is suppressed, a woman will not get normal menstrual periods. The absence of a menstrual period is called amenorrhea. While many women appreciate not having a menstrual period for the first several months after delivering a baby, breastfeeding as a form of birth control may not be completely effective. Certain conditions need to be in place for breastfeeding to contribute to preventing pregnancy.

First, a woman must breastfeed her baby up to six months of age exclusively. This means that the baby receives only breast milk; any intake of commercial infant formula or supplemental water is avoided. The baby is put to the breast to feed anytime it gives cues that it is hungry; therefore, women must breastfeed about every four hours, ideally, during the day and night. Similarly, a woman may use a breast pump to express breast milk but pumping, too, must occur at least every four hours. While women can extend the interval of feeding possibly to every six hours during the night, the expectation for exclusive breastfeeding is that feeding a baby occurs at regular intervals during the day and night.

Second, a woman must not have a menstrual period. Typically, the lack of a menstrual period signifies that ovulation is not occurring. However, some women can ovulate without having a menstrual period; pregnancy is a viable possibility for some women despite maintaining exclusive breastfeeding. The risk of pregnancy depends on the pattern of sexual activity a woman resumes following delivery of her baby. With exclusive breastfeeding, and the decreased level of estrogen that occurs with it, women often complain of vaginal dryness and a decreased sex drive, which may limit sexual activity. Rigid breastfeeding schedules coupled with caring for a newborn often leads to fatigue for a new mother, further minimizing a woman's desire or stamina for sexual activity.

Breastfeeding as a form of birth control, overall, can be about 98–99.5 percent effective. However, the method can be imperfect and unreliable due to multiple factors. A woman could easily become pregnant again soon after delivering her previous baby due to failure of breastfeeding as a method of birth control. It is recommended that women rely on breastfeeding as a birth control method only until her baby turns six months old. If a woman's menstrual period resumes, her baby begins to feed on supplemental formula, or she stops breastfeeding totally, she should use an alternative or backup method of birth control such as condoms and consult with her health-care practitioner about starting a birth control method to prevent becoming pregnant again.

20. I recently had an abortion. When can I begin using birth control?

Most birth control methods can be started immediately after an abortion. The timing of when to initiate a method depends on the type of abortion a woman had (e.g., aspiration/suction, surgical dilation and curettage or evacuation, induced, or with medication) and the type of birth control method a woman chooses. Table 1 provides guidelines for when to consider initiating birth control after an abortion.

Table 1 Timing of Birth Control Initiation Following Abortion

Birth Control Type	Aspiration/Suction, Surgical Dilatation and Curettage or Evacuation, Induced Abortion	Medication Abortion
Natural methods	**Fertility awareness methods:** may take up to three menstrual cycles for normal pattern to resume. Use a backup method (e.g., condoms)	**Fertility awareness methods:** may take up to three menstrual cycles for normal pattern to resume. Use a backup method (e.g., condoms)
Barrier methods	**Condoms:** can be used immediately when vaginal intercourse resumes **Diaphragm:** fitting for a diaphragm can occur immediately after a first-trimester abortion. After a second-trimester abortion, wait up to four weeks for a diaphragm fitting **Cervical cap:** can be used immediately when vaginal intercourse resumes	**Condoms:** can be used immediately when vaginal intercourse resumes **Diaphragm and cervical cap:** can be used as soon as vaginal intercourse resumes; often no resizing or refitting needed
Hormonal methods	**Oral contraceptive pills (OCPs), hormonal patch, or vaginal ring:** start on the day of abortion or within five days of abortion	**Oral contraceptive pills (OCPs), hormonal patch, or vaginal ring:** start on the day of abortion or within five days of abortion If bleeding is heavy, wait two to five days before using the vaginal ring

(Continued)

Table 1 (Continued)

Birth Control Type	Aspiration/Suction, Surgical Dilatation and Curettage or Evacuation, Induced Abortion	Medication Abortion
Long-acting methods	**Depo-Provera injection:** start on the day of abortion or within five days of abortion **Intrauterine device (IUD):** may be inserted immediately after an abortion procedure or at the follow-up visit post abortion Increased risk of IUD expulsion if inserted immediately after a second-trimester abortion	**Depo-Provera injection:** start on the day the abortion medication (e.g., misoprostol) is started or within five days of beginning the medication regimen **IUD:** start anytime after follow-up visit once pregnancy is confirmed terminated (i.e., the uterus is empty)
Sterilization	Can be scheduled any time after a woman decides to have the sterilization procedure	Can be scheduled any time after a woman decides to have the sterilization procedure

---

Natural (Nonhormonal) Methods

21. How does the abstinence method work?

Abstinence is considered the most natural form of birth control because it involves no medication, procedure, or product to occur. It is considered 100 percent effective because there is no chance of pregnancy occurring due to the absence of any sexual intercourse. In addition, abstinence minimizes the chance of transmitting harmful microorganisms that cause sexually transmitted diseases because no sexual activity or intercourse occurs.

Abstinence is common among people who make the conscious choice to avoid sexual contact and intercourse for moral, religious, legal, or health reasons. Abstinence, however, is one of the most troublesome forms of birth control. It works by avoiding intimacy and intercourse, which is difficult for many people since sexual arousal comes from multiple forms of stimulation. Abstinence is more than just avoiding sexual intercourse; it includes avoiding any form of sexual activity, including genital contact, and often other forms of intimacy such as caressing, massage, or bodily contact that could result in sexual arousal.

Abstinence is highly effective if people commit to following it and avoiding situations that could compromise adhering to one's abstinence plan. There are several steps individuals, or couples, can take to promote, and adhere to, abstinence. First, abstinence works only if both partners agree with observing it and communicate their feelings, expectations, and values openly with each other. Discussions, and decisions, need to occur when both people in the relationship are clearheaded and sober so a meaningful dialog can happen. It is important during these discussions to determine what sexual activities each partner can safely participate in (e.g., hugging, kissing) and identify those that trigger a strong sexual response so they can be avoided. In addition, a woman can employ natural family planning methods and identify time of increased fertility, allowing her and her partner to avoid any chance of sexual activity or arousal. It is also important for each partner to understand, and honor, the word "no" and halt any further contact or activity when that word is activated. Should sexual arousal continue, and a couple is heading inevitably toward sexual intercourse, it is best to be prepared with some form of birth control such as a barrier method like condoms. In addition, it may be necessary to consider an additional method such as emergency contraception to have as a reliable backup method should other plans fail.

22. Is using the "pull out" method safe?

The "pull out" method, also called withdrawal, is a way of preventing pregnancy by attempting to keep semen out of, and away from, the vagina. Essentially a couple has sexual intercourse, but immediately before an orgasm, a man rapidly withdraws, or "pulls out," his penis from the vagina and completes his orgasm and ejaculation outside of his partner's vagina. There are some benefits to withdrawal: it's free and always available and requires no additional products or materials to complete. However, withdrawal is difficult and is less effective than other birth control methods at preventing pregnancy.

The pull out or withdrawal method requires a man to know his body and sexual response times. Since those can both be unpredictable, withdrawal, overall, is not a reliable or effective form of birth control. For example, statistics predict that for every 100 women who use withdrawal perfectly, 4 are likely to get pregnant. That means one in four women using withdrawal will get pregnant each year. Pull out or withdrawal is discouraged as a form of birth control because of its extreme unreliability; adding another form of birth control, or using a more reliable form of birth control, is encouraged.

It is recommended that pull out or withdrawal be combined with another form of birth control, such as condoms. Withdrawal and condoms used together, for example, greatly increases the chances of preventing pregnancy. In addition, using withdrawal and having emergency contraception available will decrease the chance of pregnancy occurring if semen should get in or near the vagina.

23. How does the "rhythm" method work?

The "rhythm method," also simply called "rhythm" or the fertility awareness method, is a form of natural family planning. Rhythm relies on a woman tracking her menstrual cycle on a standard calendar and interpreting monthly bodily changes and days of menstruation to identify times of fertility or impending fertility. During those times of heightened fertility, unprotected sexual intercourse, and sexual activity, is avoided to prevent pregnancy. Conversely, a couple trying to conceive and get pregnant can use the rhythm method to identify or predict days when ovulation is most likely and determine the best days to have sex.

Using the rhythm method is simple. A woman or couple needs a basic calendar to begin to record key dates throughout a monthly menstrual cycle. In addition, there are various "apps" available for women or couples to download to a phone or computer to assist in recording key data. It is important, however, to consult with a health-care practitioner prior to initiating rhythm for birth control if a woman has just begun menstruating, recently had a baby, or stopped taking oral contraceptive pills or other forms of hormonal contraception. A woman should consult her health-care practitioner prior to initiating the rhythm method if she is breastfeeding, having irregular periods, or approaching menopause.

To begin using rhythm, a woman starts by marking any standard calendar with the first day of each menstrual period. Each day of menstrual bleeding is also recorded. Women are encouraged to also record other signs of ovulation, such as the onset of breast tenderness and changes in vaginal mucus from thick and scant to thin, more slippery, and copious, and record any changes in their overall mood. Once there are 6–12 menstrual cycles, with other physical symptoms, recorded on a calendar, a woman can begin to dissect her menstrual pattern and identify her peak times of ovulation and fertility.

First, a woman takes her calendar of data and determines the length of her menstrual cycles. She counts from the first day of menstrual bleeding or period to the first day of menstrual bleeding of her next period. The total number of those days is her menstrual cycle. For most women, this typically ranges from 28 to 35 days.

Next, a woman determines the length of her shortest menstrual cycle. Women can use a general mathematic calculation to determine their first fertile day: subtract 18 from the total number of days in the shortest cycle. For example, if the shortest cycle is 25 days long, a woman subtracts 18 from 25 (i.e., 25–18), which equals 7. In this example a woman's first day of her menstrual cycle is her first day of her period or menstrual bleeding, and her first fertile day is day 7.

A woman uses her calendar to identify her longest menstrual cycle. She counts the total days in her longest cycle and uses math again to, this time, subtract 11 from that number to determine her last fertile day in a menstrual cycle. For example, if a woman's longest cycle is 30 days long, she would subtract 11 from 30 (i.e., 30–11), which equals 19. Therefore, in this ongoing example, the first day of this woman's menstrual cycle is her first day of menstrual bleeding, her fertile time begins on day 7, and her last fertile day is day 19. Therefore, if a woman or couple is hoping to prevent pregnancy, sexual intercourse or sexual activity would be avoided, or a barrier method used, during days 7–19 of this woman's menstrual cycle. These fertile days need to be avoided at the same time each month.

There are multiple factors that can impact a woman's menstrual cycle and its regularity, including stress or illness. Therefore, women need to continue to record their monthly menstrual cycles with the calendar on an ongoing basis and update their calculations month to month. In addition, women should bring their menstrual calendars to their annual appointments with their health-care practitioner and review their calculations and additional signs of ovulation to further refine the identification of ovulation and fertile days.

Barrier Methods

24. Are condoms safe and effective?

Both male and female condoms are convenient and inexpensive and a noninvasive form of barrier method contraception, which contain no medication to prevent pregnancy and sexually transmitted diseases (STDs) from occurring when used properly and consistently. There are a variety of condoms for both men and women that can be used, which accommodate all body types. No prescription is required to obtain or use condoms. Condoms are effective at preventing pregnancy and STDs and are safe for both men and women. Thus, these factors combined make condoms the most popular form of birth control currently.

When used properly and consistently, condoms are 98 percent effective at preventing pregnancy and STDs. However, people are not perfect, and errors can occur when using condoms; typically, condoms are only about 85 percent effective overall. To minimize the impact of human error, and keep the use of condoms as effective as possible at preventing pregnancy, people must use condoms correctly with each episode of oral, vaginal, and anal sex. In addition, wearing the condom for the duration of any sexual activity, wearing it correctly, and unrolling it fully prior to initiating sexual activity enhance the condom's safety and efficacy.

The different types of condoms provide different degrees of safety and protection against pregnancy and STDs. Latex condoms are the optimal type of condom. Latex condoms have no pores, are more durable, and can withstand multiple, rigorous events of sexual activity without leaking or breakage. About 80 percent of male condoms commercially manufactured in the United States are made of latex or synthetic latex that does not contain pores. Latex works to completely block small viruses and other microorganisms that cause STDs from being transmitted from one partner to another during sexual activity; sperm is effectively blocked by latex in a condom. Natural skin, natural membrane, or lambskin condoms, in contrast, contain small pores that may permit the passage of viruses, including HIV, hepatitis B, herpes, and possibly sperm.

The manufacture of condoms is highly regulated. Industry standards partner with federal guidelines from the Food and Drug Administration and the scientific community through research to ensure condoms are safe and effective. There are strict standards in place for quality control that all condom manufacturers must adhere to before their product can reach the commercial market. To date, the condom manufacturers have not deviated from these standards and have typically exceeded the basic regulatory requirements for production. However, a well-manufactured condom will be safe and effective only if it is used properly and consistently with each episode of sexual activity.

25. There are so many different types of condoms. How do I choose the right one?

It can be overwhelming to go into any store that sells condoms. There are rows of boxes, brands, and features that are not only enticing or intriguing but also confusing. What is important to keep in mind when selecting condoms is to focus on the material the condom is made of and ignore the fancy packaging, colors, features, or designs of the various competitive brands.

The most important thing to look for when selecting a condom is the material the condom is made of. Condoms can be made of latex, polyurethane, polyisoprene, or natural animal skin like lambskin. Only latex, polyurethane, and polyisoprene are strong and nonporous enough to prevent pregnancy and the transmission of sexually transmitted diseases (STDs). If a person is not allergic to latex, it is best to use. However, if one is allergic to latex, polyurethane or polyisoprene can be used as safe substitutes. Many condoms are sold as novelty items and may not provide adequate protection against pregnancy or the transmission of STDs.

Condoms come in a variety of options. Many, for example, are colored, flavored, scented, warming, vibrating, or textured. These features are meant to enhance the experiences associated with sexual activity. However, what is intended to increase fun or the sexual experience may not afford sufficient protection against pregnancy or STDs. Some of the additional decorative features of some condoms can contribute to the development of urinary tract or vaginal infections, localized irritation, burning, or discomfort. Condoms do not need multiple decorative features to be useful; they are safe and effective in their simplest, latex form.

Both male and female condoms are individually wrapped to preserve their integrity and elasticity. A condom with a broken wrapper or one that has been exposed to air or unrolled should not be used but discarded. For men, a condom should be applied to an erect penis. The reservoir at the tip of the condom should be visible; there should be enough room at the tip of the penis to allow the condom reservoir to collect any ejaculated semen. The condom should be unrolled down the shaft or length of the penis and end at the base of the penis where the testicles or pubic hair meet the shaft of the penis. An appropriate-sized condom is one that remains snugly adhered to an erect penis and does not roll around or off the penis freely. The fit should be comfortable and not painfully tight or constrictive on any part of the penis.

Before use, a condom can be lubricated with a water-based lubricant or spermicide cream or jelly; other products like baby oil, cooking oils or vegetable shortenings, petroleum jelly, saliva, or oil-based lubricant should be avoided because they can potentially break down the integrity of a condom and cause the condom to break. The use of products other than water-based lubricants to lubricate a condom has no spermicidal effect and can cause injury or discomfort to a sex partner during sexual activity.

Once vigorous sexual activity has begun, it is important to check that the condom is still properly applied and not rolling up or loosening. If no ejaculation occurs, and the condom is still intact, additional lubricant can be applied and the condom can be used for an additional episode of sexual activity. If the condom is removed, it should never be reapplied. If ejaculation does occur, care should be taken when the penis is withdrawn from the vagina or rectum; the base of the condom should be held firmly prior to withdrawing to avoid leaking any seminal fluid and then removed and discarded.

26. How does the female condom work?

Female condoms, in contrast to the male condom, require a different approach for use because they are inserted into the vagina prior to use. Like male condoms, female condoms are individually wrapped and available in a range of sizes. The inner ring at the closed end of the sheath is used to insert the condom inside the vagina and hold it in place during sex. The rolled outer ring at the open end of the sheath remains outside the vagina and covers part of the external genitalia. To use the female condom, a small amount of water-based lubricant is applied on the outside of the closed end of the sheath. A woman can either lie down, squat, or stand with one foot up on a chair or the toilet to position herself properly to insert the condom. The inner ring at the closed end is squeezed and inserted into the vagina like the way a woman would insert a tampon. The inner ring is pushed gently into the vagina as far as it can go, typically until it reaches the cervix. As the fingers are removed from the vagina, the sheath unrolls and the outer ring hangs about an inch outside the vagina. The edges of the condom extend, or hang, over the vaginal opening, essentially forming a bag inside the vagina. When the condom is fitted properly, all surfaces of the vagina are covered.

During sexual activity or intercourse, it is normal for the female condom to move side to side; intercourse should be stopped if the penis slips between the condom and the walls of the vagina. If ejaculation has not occurred, a female condom can be gently removed from the vagina to add additional spermicide or lubricant and then reinserted into the vagina. If ejaculation occurs, the outer ring can be squeezed and twisted to contain any semen within the pouch and then gently removed from the vagina and discarded. Female condoms should not be rinsed, rerolled, or stored for future use.

While the female condom is simple to use, many women, and men, dislike the feel of the female condom and find it dampens their sexual experience. Many women dislike having to interrupt foreplay to insert the female condom or find it too messy or cumbersome to manage. The female condom cannot be used for anal sex.

27. How does the diaphragm work?

A diaphragm is a barrier method of birth control for women only. Typically made of silicone, a diaphragm is a bendable, shallow cup that is shaped like a saucer. Once inserted properly into the vagina, a diaphragm completely covers the cervix and blocks sperm from entering the cervix and potentially joining with an egg. To improve the diaphragm's effectiveness, spermicidal creams or gels are recommended to be used with a diaphragm. Spermicidal creams or gels placed inside the surface of the diaphragm aid in occluding sperm's access to the cervix by forming an additional barrier to the cervix. If random sperm should make it past the borders of the diaphragm, the spermicidal creams or gels help to slow the movement of sperm, making it more difficult for sperm to enter the cervix.

The diaphragm can be a highly effective form of birth control. However, to be completely effective, a diaphragm must be fitted correctly. A diaphragm must be used properly and consistently every time a woman has sex to prevent pregnancy. If a woman desires a diaphragm, a complete physical examination, including a pelvic examination by an experienced health-care practitioner, is required. Diaphragms come in various sizes with different strengths of tension of their outer rings depending on the manufacturer. During a pelvic examination a health-care practitioner makes several key assessments, including vaginal muscle tone, pelvic diameters, and vaginal shape. These various measurements determine the appropriate-sized diaphragm. These measurements can vary over time due to weight gain or loss, pregnancy, childbirth, or vaginal surgery. The health-care practitioner will typically write a prescription for a specific-sized diaphragm that can be filled at a pharmacy or potentially dispensed at the health-care practitioner's office.

Once the appropriate-sized diaphragm is obtained, a woman is encouraged to practice inserting and removing the diaphragm, often in the health-care practitioner's office. To insert a diaphragm, a woman first prepares the diaphragm for insertion. Holding the diaphragm in her hand with the opening upward, a woman squeezes about a teaspoon of spermicide into the cup or dome of the diaphragm. The spermicide is then spread around the surface and the rim of the diaphragm, so it is completely covered. Only spermicides are recommended; other products like petroleum jelly, other lubricants, or medicated vaginal creams can break down the integrity of the diaphragm and cause breaks or holes in the diaphragm.

The diaphragm can be inserted from several positions. It is best for a woman to lie down, squat, or stand with one leg up on a chair or the toilet. The legs, however, should be opened wide. With one hand, a woman folds the diaphragm in half, with the dome pointing down (i.e., the side containing the spermicide is facing up). The other hand holds the vagina open. The diaphragm is gently inserted into the vagina and pushed slowly inward toward the tailbone. The diaphragm should be inserted as far back into the vagina as it can go. Once inserted, the diaphragm will open. A woman then uses one finger to push the front rim of the diaphragm up behind the pubic bone toward her belly button.

To check if the diaphragm is in the correct position, a woman can use her index finger to feel her cervix through the dome of the diaphragm. The cervix should feel firm, but not bony, like the tip of her nose. If the cervix cannot be felt or if it is not covered, the diaphragm may not be in place. The diaphragm should be removed, additional spermicide applied, and reinsertion attempted. The diaphragm should not come out when a woman walks, squats, coughs, or sits. The diaphragm is in correct position when it is snugly above the pubic bone.

To be effective, a diaphragm must be used correctly with each episode of sexual intercourse. Diaphragms should not be used or left in place during a menstrual period nor should douching occur while a diaphragm is in place. A diaphragm should not be left in the vagina for more than 24 hours. After each episode of sexual activity, additional spermicide should be inserted into the vagina; the diaphragm does not need to be removed to reapply spermicide. The diaphragm, in addition, should remain in the vagina up to six hours after the last episode of sexual activity.

The diaphragm can be removed by using the index finger to grasp the rim, and gently pull it out to avoid tearing or puncturing. Once removed, the diaphragm should be washed with mild soap and water, rinsed, and allowed to air dry. The diaphragm should be stored in a cool, dry container. Prior to reusing, the diaphragm should be inspected for tears or holes (hint: fill the dome with water and look at all surfaces for leakage). If any holes or tears are found, do not use the diaphragm and opt for another method like condoms until a new diaphragm can be obtained. In addition, a woman should bring her diaphragm to her annual gynecologic appointment to allow her health-care practitioner to thoroughly inspect her diaphragm and ensure a proper fit. A diaphragm should be replaced every two years or sooner if childbirth, pelvic surgery, or a gain or loss of 15 pounds of body weight occurs.

28. Can I use spermicidal creams or lubricants safely as birth control?

Spermicide is a substance that reduces the risk of pregnancy by blocking the cervix and limiting sperm's movement. It does not kill sperm.

However, by limiting the motility or movement of sperm, the chances of sperm uniting with an egg are decreased. Sperm, in turn, can survive only a brief period of time if it does not unite with an egg. With slowed motility, the sperm eventually dies on its own.

Spermicides come in creams, gels, or suppositories. The formulation of the spermicide determines how it is used. Most commercial spermicides, however, have specific directions for use on the product or in the product packaging. Typically, using spermicide requires a woman to lie down or squat to allow access to the vagina. Using an applicator or her finger, a teaspoon-sized amount of spermicide is inserted into the vagina. After a 10-minute wait, a woman can begin sexual activity. The spermicide is typically effective for up to one hour after insertion; additional spermicide should be inserted each time a woman has sex afterward. A woman should also avoid douching for six to eight hours following her last episode of sexual intercourse.

Spermicide, while inexpensive, convenient, hormone free, and not requiring a prescription for use, is not effective as a sole form of birth control. For maximum effectiveness, the spermicide needs to completely cover the cervix which, used alone, cannot be accomplished. However, spermicide is highly effective when it is combined with another form of birth control (e.g., as a lubricant with condoms, as an additional layer of protection inside a diaphragm cup, or used in conjunction with birth control pills).

Spermicide does not reduce the risk of contracting sexually transmitted diseases. Spermicide can cause irritation to the penis or the vagina. The irritation can cause breaks or cracks in the tissue surface, thereby serving as a portal of entry for harmful, STD-causing microorganisms or the HIV virus. Care should be taken to avoid using a spermicide that causes irritation and use a brand that is less irritating.

29. What is the cervical cap, and how does it work?

A cervical cap, or simply referred to as "the cap," is another barrier method for women only. Typically made of silicone, the cervical cap is different from a diaphragm because it covers only the cervix. Where a diaphragm is a large disc that, once inside the vagina, stays snugly in place because its edges are supported against all sides of the vaginal walls, the cervical cap covers only the cervix. Women who are unable to use diaphragms often have more success using a cervical cap because it stays firmly in place directly over the cervix. The cervical cap is a smaller, sailor hat–shaped cap with a strap on one side to allow for easy removal. The cap is most effective when used with spermicide and by women who have never given birth.

Mechanism of Action

The cervical cap works, like a diaphragm, by blocking sperm from reaching the cervix. In addition, a woman uses spermicide inside the dome of the cervical cap that provides an additional layer of protection to prevent pregnancy. Since the cervical cap rests firmly against the cervix, it forms a barrier that blocks sperm from getting through to the uterus to possibly unite with an egg. If sperm cannot unite with an egg, there is no chance of pregnancy occurring, so pregnancy is impossible. Since spermicide is also used inside the cap, sperm's motility is impeded, thus further preventing pregnancy from occurring.

Benefits

There are several benefits to using the cervical cap. These include the following:

- The cervical cap is easy to use.
- Since it is a barrier method, there are no hormones, and it is safe to use while breastfeeding.
- No prescription is required to use the cervical cap in some instances.
- It can be inserted up to six hours prior to sexual activity and remain in place for up to two days after sexual activity has ceased.
- The cervical caps are sturdy and can last from 18 months to 2 years.
- Cervical caps are inexpensive.
- If a woman wants to become pregnant, she simply stops using the cervical cap.

Disadvantages

There are several disadvantages to using the cervical cap. These include the following:

- The cap cannot be used by women allergic to silicone or spermicide.
- A woman cannot use the cervical cap during her period. Women who rely on the cap as their sole source of birth control need to abstain from sex or use an alternative form of contraception during their period.

- If a woman has given birth, the size of her cervix can change. The currently available cervical caps may not fit, necessitating the need for a diaphragm or different contraceptive option.
- The cap can be difficult to insert correctly or quickly. Some women have trouble reaching far enough into the vagina to reach their cervix and apply the cap.
- The cap can be dislodged or pushed out during vigorous sexual activity, with heavy thrusting, by some sexual positions, or by penis size. Women using the cap may need to modify their sexual positions or activities to ensure the cap stays in place.
- The cap must be inserted before each episode of sexual intercourse. However, the cap can be inserted up to six hours prior to any anticipated sexual arousal or activity.
- The cap must be used with spermicide. The spermicide can be an additional cost or inconvenience for women or be a source of irritation or other unwanted side effects.
- The cap provides no protection against STDs, including HIV or Hepatitis B.

Contraindications

The cervical cap is ideal for women who have never given birth because the cervix is typically smaller and, therefore, more likely to have the cap fit snugly, and occlusive, over the cervix. However, the cap is also not indicated for women who

- have difficulty inserting the cap by themselves;
- have any anomalies or diseases of the vagina, cervix, or uterus;
- have vaginal, cervical, or uterine cancers;
- have an active vaginal or cervical infection;
- have poor vaginal muscle tone;
- have had a baby within 10–12 weeks of cap use;
- recently had surgery on the cervix;
- have a history of toxic shock syndrome.

Use

If a woman desires to use a cervical cap, she should consult with her health-care practitioner. The health-care practitioner will thoroughly review a woman's medical, surgical, menstrual, obstetrical, and sexual histories and discuss a woman's birth control options. A brief physical examination and a full pelvic examination will occur. During the pelvic exam, the health-care practitioner will assess the musculature, and tone, of the vagina, the size, shape, and density of the cervix and perform STD screenings as indicated. The health-care practitioner will determine which size cap is appropriate for a woman and advise her which size to purchase at a pharmacy. Cervical caps come in three sizes:

- Small—ideal for women who have never been pregnant or given birth
- Medium—for women who have had an abortion, miscarriage, or a Cesarean delivery
- Large—for women who have given birth vaginally in the past.

Some insurance plans may cover the purchase of the cap, so the health-care practitioner may provide a prescription for a woman to obtain one.

The health-care practitioner will instruct about how to use the cervical cap. However, it may take practice for a woman to become comfortable with using the cap. To insert a cap, a woman begins by washing her hands with soap and water. She holds the cap upside down so the domed, or cup, opening is facing up. She then puts about ¼ teaspoon of spermicide inside the cup, spreading a thin layer of spermicide on the flat part of the cap's brim. A woman then assumes a comfortable position (e.g., sitting on the edge of a chair or a toilet with her legs spread apart or standing with her foot up on a chair or the toilet or squatting on the floor) like she was inserting a tampon. A woman opens her vagina with one hand while squeezing the rim of the cap with the other. She inserts the cap into the vagina, so the side of the dome and strap is facing the vagina's opening (the long brim goes into the vagina first). The cap is then pushed deep into the vagina. Once it reaches the cervix, it stays firmly in place to cover the cervix.

The cap can be inserted up to six hours prior to the onset of sexual activity and can remain in place for up to two days after sexual activity ceases. A woman should add additional spermicide to her vagina if she is leaving the cap in place after sexual activity. The cap should stay in no longer than 48 hours.

Removing the cervical cap is easier than inserting it. The cap is equipped with a strap that allows a woman to easily grasp the cap with her fingers and pull it out. To remove the cap, a woman assumes the similar, comfortable position she used for insertion. Using her fingers, she reaches into the vagina to feel the cap at her cervix. She gently pushes against the dome to break the suction of the cap against her cervix. She then uses the same finger to loop under the strap and gently pull the cap down and out of her vagina.

Once the cap is removed, a woman washes it with soap and warm water. The cap should be allowed to air dry. No powders, baking soda, lubricants, perfumes, or alcohol should be used on the cap. It should be stored in a dry place away from extremes of cold or heat. When a woman is ready to use her cap again, she should hold the cap up to the light and inspect it for holes, tears, wrinkles, cracks, or weak spots. A woman can also fill the cap with water to test for leaks. If any leaks, tears, cracks, or holes are noted, a woman should not use the cap and use an alternative form of contraception like condoms. Caps, however, can change color or fade over time, which is normal.

Risks

The risks of using a cervical cap are related to the spermicide that is used with it. Spermicides applied inside the dome of the cap may damage the cells that line the vagina or surround the cervix. When these cells are damaged, a woman can be at increased risk for contracting an STD. Similarly, the spermicide can irritate the walls of the vagina and lead to the development of vaginal, or urinary tract, infections.

Side Effects

The most common side effect women report when using the cervical cap is vaginal irritation. Some women report increased vaginal redness, itching, burning, or discomfort following the use of the cap and spermicides. In addition, women report more frequent bladder or urinary tract infections. The cap, however, does not damage the cervix or the vaginal walls. While the cap can be dislodged or fall out during vigorous sexual activity, it will not get lost within the vagina nor become irretrievable if it gets displaced.

30. What is the contraceptive sponge, and how does it work?

The contraceptive sponge, also called the "sponge" or, by the most familiar commercial brand, the "Today Sponge," is another form of barrier contraception available to women. The sponge is a soft, two-inch, disc-shaped device made of polyurethane foam that contains a spermicide and a small loop of nylon fabric to assist with removal. The sponge is inserted into the vagina before sex to prevent pregnancy. The sponge works in two ways: it covers the cervix to prevent any sperm from entering the uterus, and it contains spermicide that impedes sperm's motility, making it impossible for sperm to reach an egg. The sponge can be used by itself, or it can be used along with condoms to provide an additional layer of protection against pregnancy, sexually transmitted diseases (STDs), and HIV.

The sponge, when used properly and consistently, is about 91 percent effective. The sponge is more effective when used by women who have never given birth. The sponge, however, provides no protection against STDs or HIV. The spermicide in the sponge (typically Nonoxynol-9) can irritate the vagina and make it easier for the harmful microorganisms that cause STDs to enter a woman's body. Using the sponge with condoms provides protection against both pregnancy and STDs.

Mechanism of Action

The sponge contains spermicide that gets activated immediately prior to insertion. A woman sprinkles water onto the sponge to activate the spermicide. Once the sponge is inserted deep into the vagina, it fits snugly against the cervix to completely occlude the opening to the uterus. With the cervix blocked, sperm cannot enter the uterus to potentially unite with an egg. Since the sponge contains spermicide, sperm's movement is impeded, making it harder for sperm to swim toward the cervix. Sperm has a limited lifespan, so if it does not reach an egg, it will die.

The sponge begins to work as soon as it's activated with water and inserted into the vagina. The sponge can be inserted up to 24 hours before sex. A woman can take her time to carefully insert the sponge before the onset of sexual activity, and she does not have to interrupt progressive foreplay to insert the device. Once the sponge is inserted, a woman can have multiple episodes of sex over 24 hours without having to replace the sponge. Unlike the cervical cap, the sponge is less likely to get dislodged by vigorous sexual activity or certain sexual positions. The sponge, however, needs to stay in place for at least 6 hours after sex but should not stay in the vagina for more than 30 hours total. The sponge does not have to stay in the vagina for a full 30 hours. However, for full contraceptive benefit, the sponge needs to remain in place for at least six hours after the last episode of sex.

Benefits

There are several benefits of the sponge. These include the following:

- The sponge is hormone free and is safe to use while breastfeeding.
- No prescription is needed to use the sponge.

- The sponge is inexpensive.
- The sponge is available over the counter at most drug stores or through online retailers.
- The sponge is small and individually wrapped to allow it to fit easily in a pocket or a bag.
- Protection against pregnancy is for 24 hours.
- It is effective immediately.
- No impact on future fertility—the sponge stops working immediately once it's removed.
- There is no interruption of foreplay or sex because the sponge is inserted up to six hours prior to sexual activity.
- A woman will not feel the sponge inside her vagina, and her male partners will not notice or feel the sponge during sex.

Disadvantages

Several disadvantages exist with the sponge also. These include the following:

- The sponge needs to be used properly each time.
- The sponge can be difficult to insert and takes practice to get fully comfortable using it.
- The sponge can be difficult to remove.
- The sponge is not reusable, and a new sponge is needed for all future sexual activity.
- The sponge does not protect against STDs or HIV.
- The spermicide in the sponge can cause vaginal irritation and predispose a woman to contracting an STD.
- Using the sponge increases the risk of toxic shock syndrome (TSS).
- The sponge can be wet and messy.
- The sponge can absorb natural vaginal moisture and make sex dry and uncomfortable.

Use

The sponge does not require a prescription, nor does it require a physical or pelvic examination from a health-care practitioner. In the United States, the sponge is available in retail pharmacies, some supermarkets, online at the Today Sponge's website, or through other online retailers that sell barrier contraceptives like condoms. The sponge comes in only one size that fits most women. The sponge is also inexpensive, costing approximately $10–15 depending on where it's sold.

After a woman purchases the sponge, she inserts the sponge like the way she would insert a tampon. First, a woman washes her hands with soap and water. The sponge is removed from its wrapper and then moistened, or activated, with about one tablespoon of water. Once moistened, a woman gently squeezes the sponge until she sees suds (it needs to be totally wet, but not saturated, to activate the spermicide). The sponge should not be squeezed too much nor made dry; it should be wet and foamy at the time of insertion.

With the indented side of the sponge facing up, a woman folds the sides upward (i.e., away from the nylon loop) until the sponge is long and narrow. It is important that the indented side is facing the front side of a woman's body and the nylon loop is facing her rectum or the back side of her body.

A woman can either sit on the toilet with her legs apart, squat on the floor, or stand with one foot up on the toilet or on a chair. Using her opposite hand to gently open her vagina, a woman slowly slides the sponge deep into her vagina and pushes it as far back as she can with her fingers. Once a woman lets go of the sponge, it will unfold and open to cover her cervix.

Once the sponge is in place, it is important that a woman check the placement of the sponge to ensure it's in proper position. A woman gently inserts her finger into her vagina and points it back toward her cervix until she can feel the edge of the sponge. She should sweep around the edges of the sponge to ensure that her cervix is completely covered. She should be able to feel the nylon loop on the bottom of the sponge. Once a woman verifies her cervix is covered, she is protected against pregnancy for the next 24 hours.

To remove the sponge, a woman again washes her hands with soap and water. She will slide a clean finger inside her vagina and hook it around the nylon loops of the sponge. Once grasped, she will gently glide the sponge out of her vagina. If a woman cannot grasp the nylon loop, she can attempt to grasp the sponge itself and pull it out of her vagina. If a woman has difficulty reaching the sponge, she uses her vaginal muscles to bear down (like she was going to the bathroom) while reaching for the sponge.

The used sponge should be discarded into the trash. Used sponges should not be flushed down the toilet. Sponges are not reusable, nor can they be taken out and put back in multiple times. Once the sponge is removed, it should be discarded.

Risk and Side Effects

The risks and side effects of the sponge are the same. These include the following:

- Vaginal irritation and increased vaginal dryness
- Increased incidence of urinary tract or vaginal infections
- Increased risk of STDs
- Increased risk of TSS

Contraceptive Pills

31. How do oral contraceptive pills work?

Since their introduction in the 1960s, oral contraceptive pills (OCPs) have evolved into a safe, reliable form of birth control for women. For more than four decades women have been able to have control over the timing of when to become pregnant or to not have children at all. Women can also enjoy sexual activity while using OCPs because the chance of pregnancy is minimized with the proper and consistent use of prescribed OCPs. While there are several different formulations of OCPs, what makes OCPs effective is the combination of estrogen and progesterone or their synthetic derivatives. OCPs come in a variety of formulations: progesterone-only, estrogen-only, and, the most common, a pill that contains a combination of estrogen and progesterone. OCPs work by directly influencing the feedback mechanism of a woman's endocrine system. The feedback mechanism, and the interference of the closed loop by synthetic hormones, is how OCPs work to prevent pregnancy.

Progestin-Only OCPs

The progesterone (or progestin)-only OCP, often called the "mini pill" because it contains no estrogen, contains a significantly lower dose of progestin compared to the combined OCPs (typically 0.35 mg). Currently, the drug norethindrone is the leading progestin used in mini pill formulations. The primary action of the progestin-only pill is to prevent pregnancy by causing the cervical mucus to thicken, thereby impeding the ability of sperm cells to reach an egg for fertilization. Progestin-only pills also stop ovulation.

Progestin-only pills come in a pack of 28 tablets, each containing the same amount of progestin. It is important that a pill be taken each day at the same time to maintain the maximum effectiveness of the drug.

Estrogen-Only OCPs

It is rare to use OCPs that contain only estrogen because of the potential side effects estrogen used alone can cause in a woman's body. However, it is still a key component of OCPs. In OCPs, the dose of estrogen is typically 25–50 micrograms per pill. Synthetic estrogens in an OCP work by interfering with the natural endocrine system feedback mechanism between a woman's brain and her ovaries. Synthetic estrogen in an OCP stops the pituitary gland from producing the two key hormones needed for ovulation: follicle-stimulating hormone (FSH) and luteinizing hormone (LH). Therefore, ovulation is prevented. Because the feedback mechanism is interrupted, cervical mucus production is altered and becomes thicker, like the effect of progesterone. The thicker cervical mucus makes it more difficult for sperm to travel toward an egg. In addition, the synthetic estrogen causes the uterine lining to fail to grow and thicken, making it further unfavorable for a fertilized egg to implant and grow. However, estrogen alone, while beneficial to preventing pregnancy, can also cause damage and cellular changes of the uterine lining or ovaries when taken repeatedly over time. To help minimize any negative cellular changes to the cells of the uterus, to prevent uterine cancers, and to enhance the ability of OCPs to prevent pregnancy, estrogen is typically combined with progesterone.

Estrogen and Progesterone in OCPs

OCPs work best when used as a combination of estrogen and progesterone. These two hormones, when combined, interfere with the feedback mechanism between a woman's pituitary gland and the ovaries that causes the following effects (Table 2):

Table 2 Effects of Estrogen and Progesterone in OCPs

Estrogen	Progesterone
Prevents the pituitary gland from producing FSH and LH, so ovulation does not occur	Stops LH production in the pituitary gland, so no egg is released
	Limits the ability of an egg to be fertilized by sperm
	Causes changes to the uterine lining, making it harder for a fertilized egg to implant
	Causes the cervical mucus to thicken, hindering the ability of sperm to travel toward, or reach, an egg for fertilization

The dosage of each hormone within the combined OCPs varies. Typical doses of hormones in a combined OCP are 20–35 micrograms of estrogen or its synthetic derivatives, and 0.35 mg of a progestin. For years, combined OCPs contained the same amount of estrogen and progesterone in each pill that was taken each day. Over time, multiple side effects and significant medical complications were reported. To minimize these undesired side effects and complications, the "phasic" approach was introduced for dosing OCPs.

The phasic approach allows the amounts of estrogen, progesterone, or both to be altered over the course of a monthly cycle or within each pack of pills per month. The phasic approach includes pills that are

1. biphasic—two different doses of the hormones exist within the pack of pills;
2. triphasic—three different doses of the hormones exist within the pack of pills taken over the course of a month;
3. quadraphasic—four different doses of the hormones exist within the pack of pills taken over the course of a month.

Current formulations of OCPs on the market allow for two different phasic approaches:

1. Progesterone levels change throughout the pill cycle, but the estrogen level remains the same in all the pills throughout a pill cycle.
2. Both the progesterone and estrogen levels change during the pill cycle.

Regardless of the phasic approach or formulation used, the common practice is to begin with the lowest dose of each hormone possible and then adjust as needed (i.e., increase or decrease the amount of either estrogen or progesterone contained within a pill by discontinuing one formulation and beginning or using another) based on side effects a woman may experience or report. A woman's primary responsibility with OCPs is to take a pill, each day, by mouth, as prescribed.

32. How do I start taking OCPs, and what should I do if I miss pills?

Oral contraceptive pills (OCPs), or birth control pills, are a convenient form of contraception because a typical regimen involves a woman taking only one pill each day for full protection. Regardless of the formulation (e.g., progestin-only or combined estrogen and progesterone pills), a woman has three options for beginning OCPs:

1. *First day of period start.* A woman obtains a prescription from a healthcare provider and takes the first pill in her monthly pack on the first day of her menstrual period. By starting on the first day of a period, a woman does not need to use a backup method of pregnancy protection like condoms because the OCPs will be effective at preventing pregnancy before the time she ovulates next or becomes fertile.
2. *Quick start.* This option allows a woman to begin to start her monthly pill pack immediately after obtaining a prescription for the OCPs and as soon as she receives her first monthly pack of pills, regardless of when her period is. Starting OCPs this way is convenient, but the ability of the OCPs to prevent pregnancy is less effective during the initial month. A backup form of contraception (e.g., condoms, diaphragm, abstinence) is needed for at least 7–10 days following a quick start initiation of pills.
3. *Sunday start.* With this option a woman takes her first pill from a monthly pill pack on the first Sunday following the start of her menstrual period. If a woman's period starts on a Sunday, then she starts her pill that day. Like the quick start option, the ability of the OCPs to prevent pregnancy is not fully effective for several days, so a backup method of pregnancy protection (e.g., condoms, abstinence) is required for at least 7–10 days following initiation.

Regardless of what schedule a woman uses to start taking OCPs, there are general guidelines she needs to follow to improve the likelihood that the OCPs will be effective toward preventing pregnancy:

1. Take one (1) pill every day at the same time each day. This helps establish a pattern and makes daily pill taking a habit. It also keeps

the level of hormones consistent within a woman's body and avoids prolonged periods of low or inadequate hormone levels.

2. Take pills in the monthly pack from left to right, beginning with the pill in the upper left corner of the first row and ending the month (or cycle) with the last pill in the last row in the lower right corner.
3. If the monthly pill pack has hormone-free or placebo pills at the end, continue to take those pills on the same schedule as the others.
4. When the last pill in the monthly pack is taken, start a new monthly pack the next day.

If a woman takes her required dose of OCP daily (i.e., she does not miss a dose), she is protected from pregnancy each month. However, multiple circumstances can impact a woman's ability to take her OCP each day. Missing a dose of an OCP does not automatically mean she is unprotected against pregnancy; the number of doses missed or the number of days that elapse between doses determines if a current month's pack of pills is still effective to prevent pregnancy. The general rule for women to follow is to never take fewer than 21 consecutive (or active) pills and never have more than seven consecutive pill-free days. Backup methods like condoms, diaphragms, or abstinence can be used to provide protection against pregnancy if doses of OCPs are missed or lapsing or if a monthly OCP pack was started late.

The chance of pregnancy depends not only on how many pills were missed but also on when those pills were missed within a monthly pill pack or cycle. This risk of pregnancy is greatest when the active or hormonal pills are missed, or at the end of the active pills when the hormone-free interval is the longest. Table 3 can be used as a guide for managing missed pills (combined OCPs and progestin-only OCPs) during a monthly cycle or pill pack:

Table 3 Managing Missed OCPs

Issue	Actions
One (1) combined OCP is missed or taken late (or a new pack started late)	– A woman should take the pill she missed as soon as she remembers and then take the next dose at the regularly scheduled time (it is possible that a woman may be taking two pills on the same day, one at the time she remembers and then a pill at the regular time) – To remain fully protected against pregnancy, a woman should use a backup method like condoms, diaphragm, or abstinence for at least a week (seven days) after missing a pill dose

(Continued)

Table 3 (Continued)

Issue	Actions
More than one (1) combined OCP missed	– Protection against pregnancy depends on how much hormone was missed. If a woman misses the hormone-free or placebo pills, her chances of pregnancy are minimal. However, most women miss doses of OCPs that contain hormone (e.g., estrogen) 1. *If two active (or hormone) pills are missed*: take the missed pills as soon as possible and then continue taking your next pill on schedule daily (both missed pills can be taken at the same time on the same day) 2. *If the missed pills were in the third week of the monthly pill pack*: a woman should continue taking the active (or hormone) pills in the current pack daily. However, once the active pills are done, a woman should discard the pack (and remaining pills) and immediately begin a new pack (i.e., the inactive, placebo, or hormone-free pills should not be taken but discarded)
If pill(s) were missed during the first week and unprotected sex occurred	– A woman should use emergency contraception (e.g., Plan B) for maximum protection in addition to taking the next scheduled dose
If a woman misses a dose of progestin-only OCP	– A woman should take the missed dose as soon as she remembers it and go back to taking progestin-only contraceptives at her regular scheduled time – If the pill is more than 3 hours late, a woman should use a backup method of birth control for the next 48 hours – If a woman is not sure what to do about the pills she has missed, she should keep taking progestin-only contraceptives and use a backup method of birth control until she speaks to her health-care practitioner

The inconsistent use of OCPs is a major reason for unintended pregnancy. A woman who frequently misses pills should consider alternate contraceptive methods or use a different method entirely when taking pills daily becomes difficult.

33. Can I stop taking OCPs at any time if I want to become pregnant?

It is important to remember that oral contraceptive pills (OCPs) do not affect a woman's fertility; rather, they impede or reduce her ability to become pregnant. Therefore, once a woman stops using OCPs, her level of fertility is unchanged. Her ability to become pregnant should also return to whatever it was prior to initiating OCPs. For example, if a woman had irregular periods prior to initiating OCPs, she will most likely resume irregular periods once she stops taking OCPs. Similarly, a woman who had no-fail, 28-day cycles prior to starting OCPs should expect the same menstrual regularity to return when she stops using OCPs. While there is a good chance a woman could conceive within the first month after stopping OCPs, a woman needs to understand that becoming pregnant could take several months, especially if she had irregular menstrual cycles previously.

Women can opt to stop using OCPs at any time if they wish to become pregnant. However, simply stopping the use of OCPs does not mean a woman will instantly become pregnant with her next ovulation. While some women have become pregnant immediately after stopping OCPs, other factors can impact a woman's ability to become pregnant. Each woman is unique; it could take months, or several menstrual cycles, for ovulation to resume or monthly menstrual periods to return to normal.

Although a woman may be tempted to stop OCPs at any time, abruptly stopping pills or discontinuing them randomly at any time within a monthly cycle is not recommended. Since OCPs are essentially made of synthetic hormones, stopping OCPs randomly or abruptly throws off the balance of hormones in a woman's body, which can lead to mood swings, irritability, irregular bleeding, sleep disturbances, or other bodily symptoms. Therefore, it is recommended that a woman taper off her OCPs by completing the full monthly pack, including any placebo or hormone-free pills, and go through her normal monthly menstrual period. When her period is over, a woman would not start a new pack of OCPs. She would continue to have normal monthly menstrual cycles thereafter unless she becomes pregnant.

After discontinuing the use of OCPs, a woman's period can show up at any time within the next few days, weeks, or months. It is not uncommon for a woman to go several weeks without a menstrual period or to have intermittent, irregular spotting. However, despite irregular periods or spotting, a woman is still likely to continue to ovulate about two weeks before any bleeding is seen. Since the likelihood of menstrual irregularity or spotting is high, it is recommended that women "wait a cycle." This means that a woman would stop taking her OCPs and then wait until she has completed one (or possibly two) complete menstrual cycles before trying to conceive. While waiting one or two cycles may interfere with a woman's plan to become pregnant immediately, doing so will allow her to identify the physical signs that she is ovulating, such as breast tenderness, mood changes, or changes in the character or consistency of her vaginal mucus. Recognizing the onset of these symptoms assists a woman to determine her most fertile days of the month and increase her chances of becoming pregnant. Since the process of stopping OCPs can be complex overall, it is recommended that a woman see her health-care practitioner for a preconception visit.

A preconception visit occurs before a woman becomes pregnant. Since 50 percent of all pregnancies are unintended, meaning a baby is developing weeks before a woman realizes or discovers she is pregnant, the preconception visit ensures that a woman, or a couple, is as healthy and prepared as possible for safe, and successful, conception. During the preconception visit, a woman or couple can expect the following:

1. *Medical history review.* Even if a woman is already known to the health-care practitioner, a thorough review of her medical and surgical history will take place. Her family history will be reviewed to look for any hereditary diseases or genetic disorders that may require screening tests before, or immediately after, becoming pregnant. This is also when all medications taken will be reviewed, including any herbal or vitamin supplements and over-the-counter preparations.
2. *Gynecologic history review.* The health-care practitioner will carefully review a woman's sexual and reproductive history. Specifically, previous pregnancies, births, miscarriages, abortions, or sexually transmitted diseases (STDs) will be carefully reviewed. A detailed description of a woman's current menstrual cycle will also occur to capture the current length of her cycles, amount and duration of bleeding, and any obvious symptoms of ovulation.
3. *Lifestyle assessment.* The health-care practitioner will ask targeted questions about a woman's, or couple's, lifestyle. Specifically, smoking and use of tobacco products, alcohol, and recreational drugs will be

thoroughly explored. A woman may be asked questions about her job to see if there are any potential exposures to toxic substances or safety hazards that could impact conception or sustaining a pregnancy. Nutrition, exercise, and sleep habits are also reviewed.

4. *Physical and gynecologic examinations.* The health-care practitioner will want to perform a physical exam to determine a woman's current state of health and readiness for conception and pregnancy. A gynecologic exam may be performed if a woman is due for a Pap test or requires any STD screenings. A breast exam may be included.

5. *Laboratory testing.* The health-care practitioner will combine any findings from the medical history review and the physical exam to determine if any laboratory blood tests are needed. For example, if blood tests are not previously done, the health-care practitioner may test a woman's immunity to diseases, such as measles, mumps, rubella, or varicella (the virus that causes chicken pox). Each of these diseases could cause significant harm to a fetus or lead to a miscarriage. Additional tests could include measuring a woman's vitamin D levels, thyroid function, and levels of iron and hemoglobin in her blood or determining her blood type and Rh factor.

6. *Planning.* This is a time for a woman or couple to ask questions and have an open conversation with the health-care practitioner. The health-care practitioner will create an individualized plan for each woman. Specifically, the health-care practitioner will outline how and when a woman should stop taking OCPs. The health-care practitioner will also review the menstrual cycle and assist a woman to identify when her fertile time is within each cycle and to identify some of the physical changes that occur during those fertile times. There is often a discussion about the use of home pregnancy tests, interpreting the results or when to seek follow-up.

Most women will receive a prescription for prenatal vitamins if they have not already begun them. Prenatal vitamins contain folic acid, which is a necessary form of an essential B vitamin. Folic acid helps prevent neural tube defects such as spina bifida or anencephaly during the early stages of fetal development. Women will also receive nutrition information about maintaining a healthy weight and diet and how to limit caffeine and alcohol intake. Women who smoke will be advised to quit and receive information on smoking cessation. Women will also be encouraged to exercise and explore alternative modalities like yoga and meditation that have been implicated to enhance fertility. Finally, a woman will be advised about when to follow up with the health-care practitioner for test results or for eventual prenatal care.

34. Do I use the same pill all the time? Will I ever need to change the type of pill I use?

A variety of oral contraceptive pills (OCPs) exist for a health-care practitioner to prescribe, with over 30 different brands available in the United States. While many of these brands contain similar hormones and doses, there are multiple formulations for a health-care practitioner to choose from and prescribe. Combined OCPs, the most common form of birth control pill used, contain an estrogen component (e.g., ethinyl estradiol, mestranol, or estradiol) and a progesterone component (e.g., levonorgestrel, desogestrel, or drospirenone). The formulation of OCP prescribed depends on several factors, including a woman's individual risk factors for dangerous side effects like blood clots, medical history, preferences, cost, and the health-care practitioner's recommendations for specific formulations or brands.

Health-care practitioners typically opt to start a woman on the lowest dose of estrogen possible. Because research has demonstrated that using lower doses of estrogen are equally as effective at preventing pregnancy while also minimizing some unfavorable side effects like nausea, headaches, and breast tenderness, formulations of OCPs now come in low dose (35 micrograms of estrogen or less) and ultralow dose (20 micrograms of estrogen or less).

Since most women are on the lowest possible dose of estrogen when using a combined OCP, and complications from these OCPs are less common, a woman could remain on the same brand and formulation of OCP for a prolonged or extended period of time. Changing OCPs is not necessary. However, some situations could require a woman to change her brand or formulation of OCP.

Women receive education from a health-care practitioner when starting OCPs, which emphasizes monitoring for signs and symptoms like chest pain, shortness of breath, frequent or unrelenting headaches, leg pain, or swelling. The presence of these symptoms after starting OCPs, or at any time during their use, would warrant stopping the current formulation of OCP and changing to a different brand or formulation (or stopping the use of OCPs entirely in some situations).

Other side effects are less serious but could also cause a woman to change her brand or formulation of OCP. The most common side effect women experience with OCPs is menstrual irregularity, including breakthrough bleeding, spotting, or missed periods. Often a change in the dose of estrogen in the OCP can minimize and regulate irregular bleeding.

Other symptoms like nausea, weight gain, headaches, mood changes, or decreased libido can be adjusted by lowering the estrogen dose or changing the brand of OCP. Some women, conversely, may opt to change pills so they can harness the benefits of other formulations like extended-cycle pills. Women can also opt to come off OCPs entirely in favor of other birth control methods.

If a woman needs to change the brand or formulation of OCP she is currently on, there are several ways she can safely do it (Table 4).

Table 4 Changing OCPs

Option	Notes
1. Finish the entire pack of pills she is currently taking (including any placebo or hormone-free pills)	– Instead of beginning a new pack of the same pills, a woman begins the new brand or formulation pill pack – For maximum protection against pregnancy, a woman may be advised to use a backup method like condoms or abstinence for several days or for a full menstrual cycle
2. Start a new brand or formulation at any time during a cycle	– Menstrual irregularity may continue, and certain formulations may not be immediately effective – A backup method like condoms or abstaining from sex should be used for several days or a full menstrual cycle
3. If switching from a combined OCP to a progestin-only pill, a woman can switch pills at any time	– A woman should use a backup method like condoms or abstain from sex for several days for maximum protection against pregnancy
4. If switching from a progestin-only pill to a combined OCP, a woman can begin taking her combined OCP at any time	– There is no need to wait for the next menstrual period to begin – A woman should use a backup method like condoms or abstain from sex for several days for maximum protection against pregnancy

35. How might my periods change while I am on birth control pills?

One of the primary benefits of using oral contraceptive pills (OCPs) is the improvement women experience in monthly menstrual periods. Women report shorter, lighter, monthly menstrual periods or no monthly period at all while on OCPs. OCPs are designed to prevent pregnancy in two ways: to interfere with a woman's natural endocrine feedback mechanism and suppress ovulation, and to cause changes within the uterus that make it difficult for a sperm to reach an egg while making the uterus inhospitable toward a fertilized egg implanting. When a woman is not using OCPs, her body goes through natural fluctuations in the level of reproductive hormones from within her endocrine system that prepare her body for releasing an egg. Therefore, if a woman is taking her OCP properly and consistently, she should not ovulate.

Similarly, the hormones in combined OCPs stop the growth of the endometrium, or inner lining of the uterus, that would accept and nourish a fertilized egg. In a normal menstrual period when OCPs are not being used, the sudden drop in hormone levels causes the endometrium to shed, which is the typical monthly menstrual bleeding. While on OCPs, the endometrium is absent. The bleeding a woman experiences is not true menstrual bleeding; instead, it is withdrawal bleeding that the uterus undergoes when it is suddenly deprived of regular doses of estrogen in the OCP.

Each woman will have different bleeding patterns while on OCPs depending on the type of OCP she is taking. For example, a woman taking a 21/7 monophasic pack of pills will have a steady dose of estrogen for 21 days and then placebo or hormone-free pills for 7 days. During the final seven days, a woman will have her "period" of predictable bleeding, which can start on day 2 or 3 of the placebo pills and last three to five days until the next pack of pills containing hormones begins. Some women may have only one day of light bleeding or have slight, sporadic, pink spotting only. Conversely, some women have no bleeding or spotting at all while on OCPs.

The absence of bleeding, or a lighter episode of monthly bleeding, is normal while on OCPs. However, some women may experience erratic episodes of bleeding like breakthrough bleeding or persistent spotting. This erratic bleeding does not mean the OCPs are not working, but it can be an inconvenience for most women. This kind of bleeding can occur if doses of OCP are missed or if the dose of estrogen in the OCP is too low.

A health-care practitioner can evaluate the bleeding and revise the OCP formulation, brand or schedule.

However, if vaginal bleeding becomes excessive, a woman needs to consult her health-care practitioner. Bleeding that is bright red, copious, and saturating two to five sanitary pads per hour requires immediate attention, even if a woman is on OCPs. Similarly, if a woman is passing clots, especially ones that are greater than an inch in diameter, she should be evaluated. Heavy vaginal bleeding that is accompanied by fever, abdominal pain, severe cramping, back pain, or vaginal discharge should be evaluated by a health-care practitioner immediately or in an emergency department (Table 5).

Table 5 Bleeding Patterns while on OCPs

Type of Bleeding	Significance
Bleeding in the first three months of starting OCPs or a new OCP	– This is typically normal – The lining of the uterus must adjust to the stimulation from new levels of estrogen and progesterone – It can take one to two packs of pills or cycles to regulate
Bleeding after missing a dose or more of OCP	– This is typically normal – If a dose of OCP is missed, it might cause sudden withdrawal bleeding – It can take several days to reregulate once the missed dose has been taken and a woman resumes her normal pill schedule
Lighter menstrual periods while on OCPs	– This is typically normal – The lower doses of estrogen and progesterone in a combined OCP keep the uterine lining thin, so periods are shorter and lighter
Bleeding after long-term OCP use	– This is typically *not* normal – First, determine if doses were missed – Anything that alters the absorption or clearance of the OCP like an intestinal virus, vomiting, vigorous exercise, certain medications or fever can render the OCP ineffective and cause unexpected bleeding

36. What do I need to look out for while I am taking OCPs?

The variety of oral contraceptive pills (OCPs) available today contains varying amounts of estrogen, progesterone, or their derivatives. While most OCPs use the lowest amounts of hormones possible, different preparations that offer higher and lower doses of both hormones are on the market, so health-care practitioners have a variety of options to choose from to meet a woman's individual needs. Overall, however, the formulations of OCPs are safe. However, the hormones in OCPs are meant to purposely raise a woman's levels of estrogen, progesterone, or both to unnatural levels. These hormones, while targeted to suppress ovulation and exert an effect on the tissues of the uterus, also exert an impact on other areas of the body, such as the breasts, clotting factors, the gastrointestinal (GI) tract, or the brain. Because OCPs can affect several body systems, women may experience benign side effects or ones that require immediate medical attention from a health-care practitioner.

When a woman begins OCPs, she is given extensive education about how to use her OCPs and the warning signs she needs to constantly monitor for. OCPs do not cause clots to form; they do, however, support their development. Because estrogen causes an increase in the blood plasma's concentration of clotting factors II, VII, VIII, X, XII and fibrinogen, a woman is potentially at a higher risk for blood clots to form. In addition, if the OCP is a combination of estrogen and progesterone, the progesterone component is believed to support or enhance estrogen's ability to increase the concentration of those clotting factors. Because the formation of blood clots (or venous thromboemboli) is a potential risk, a woman taking OCPs is educated to monitor for "ACHES," an acronym for serious side effects:

A: Abdominal pain. While not directly related to clotting, a woman on OCPs is at risk for an unintended pregnancy, tubal or ectopic pregnancy, ruptured or enlarging ovarian cysts, or ruptured liver tumor.

C: Chest pain. Sharp, crushing chest pain or heaviness could be indicative of a clot occluding one of the major cardiac vessels or signaling a heart attack (i.e., myocardial infarction) occurring. Similarly, chest pain that occurs with breathing, a persistent cough, and the presence of bloody or blood-tinged phlegm could signal a clot in the pulmonary vasculature (i.e., pulmonary embolism).

H: Headaches that are intense, or accompanied by vomiting, dizziness, fainting, weakness, or numbness to an arm, leg, or entire side of the body, could signal a clot in the cerebral vasculature of the brain (or a "stroke").

E: Eye problems. Visual changes like blurred vision, flashing lights, and partial or complete visual loss could signal a clot in the ocular vasculature.

S: Sudden leg pain, swelling, or redness of the calf, thigh, or entire leg could signal a clot in the vasculature of the leg. Similar symptoms can occur in the arm also.

Women are instructed to notify their health-care practitioner, or go to the emergency department, immediately if any of these symptoms occur. However, there are less emergent symptoms women need to monitor for and communicate to their health-care practitioner if they occur. These include the following:

1. *Nausea.* This is often the first, and most common, symptom women experience when starting OCPs. Nausea can last up to three months after initiating OCPs and may be relieved if a woman takes her OCP with food and not on an empty stomach. Persistent nausea, however, should be reported to a health-care practitioner for further evaluation.

2. *Mood changes.* Many women report new or heightened feelings of depression while on OCPs. Estrogen in OCPs acts on specific centers in the brain that can cause changes in mood. Persistent feelings of depression, or a wide, unpredictable pattern of mood swings, should be reported to the health-care practitioner.

3. *Breast tenderness or soreness.* The tissues of the breast are highly receptive to estrogen. OCPs can cause the breasts to enlarge and stay sensitive, or ache. It is recommended that women limit caffeine and salt intake if this occurs and wear a soft, fully supportive bra. Follow-up with a health-care practitioner is recommended to thoroughly evaluate the breasts.

4. *Headaches.* Mild, sporadic headaches are common while a woman is taking OCPs, but they are often relieved by over-the-counter analgesics like acetaminophen or ibuprofen. However, a headache that is unrelenting and associated with dizziness, weakness (especially of an arm, leg, or entire side of a body), or vomiting requires immediate medical attention.

5. *Spotting between periods.* Up to 50 percent of women report some form of menstrual irregularity when initiating OCPs, including irregular periods or, more commonly, spotting or bleeding between periods. Menstrual irregularity should resolve and stabilize within three to six months after starting OCPs; however, it should be reported to the health-care practitioner at follow-up visits.

6. *Missed periods.* Some women may skip periods depending on the formulation and schedule of their OCPs. Also, illness, stress, or travel with changes to time zones, the body clock, or sleep cycles could contribute to missed periods. A woman should still consult her health-care practitioner if two periods are missed despite proper and consistent use of OCPs.

7. *Vaginal discharge.* OCPs can cause a woman to have increased vaginal lubrication or, the opposite, reports of increased vaginal dryness. Both are normal, but if the increased discharge becomes too excessive, foul smelling, colored green, yellow or brown, or irritating, a woman should notify her health-care practitioner. Similarly, if vaginal dryness becomes irritating, or causes sex, sitting, or walking to become painful, the health-care practitioner should be notified.

8. *Weight gain.* The hormones in OCPs often cause fluid retention, especially in the breasts, hips, or abdominal areas that contribute to weight gain. Significant weight gain, or the persistent inability to lose weight, should be discussed with a health-care practitioner.

9. *Bloating and gas.* Estrogen causes fluid retention, while progesterone slows motility of the intestines, leading to gas and bloating. While these symptoms can be relieved with modifications in diet, water intake, or exercise, they should be discussed with a health-care practitioner if they are persistent and do not change due to any modifications in diet or exercise.

10. *Skin changes.* Because OCPs block testosterone, many women will report improvements in acne, skin redness, or outbreaks of pimples like white or black heads. However, on OCPs, women may notice an increase in acne, brown spots, or pigmentation to the skin. Also, women may notice increased redness to the cheeks, forehead, or across the nasal bridge. The health-care practitioner will evaluate if there are any immediate, or secondary, medical conditions occurring or if referral to a specialist, such as a dermatologist, is warranted.

11. *Vaginal infections.* OCPs do not cause vaginal infections, but they can contribute to a decrease in the normal bacterial flora found in the GI tract and in the vagina. Long-term use of OCPs could, therefore, contribute to vaginal yeast infections or possibly bacterial vaginosis. It is important for women who use OCPs and are sexually active to monitor for any changes in vaginal discharge or odor, or for the onset of pain or discomfort, so they can be properly evaluated and screened by a health-care practitioner.

37. Are there foods or medications that interfere with OCPs?

Oral contraceptive pills (OCPs), like any other type of prescription medication, can interact with food, other prescription medications, over-the-counter medications, or vitamin and herbal supplements. It is important to learn what foods or medications can interact with OCPs because most of the interactions tend to weaken one medication or the other. There is a chance for an OCP to be weakened or ineffective in the presence of some other prescription medications or herbal supplements.

Food is less likely to have an impact on OCPs. However, there is an ongoing belief that certain foods like licorice, yam, soy, or dairy products could impair the effectiveness of OCPs.

- Licorice can raise blood pressure but also exerts an effect on reproductive hormones. While licorice eaten in small quantities is harmless, large amounts or daily consumption over time could diminish the effectiveness of OCPs and lead to unplanned pregnancy.
- For many generations, wild yam was believed to promote fertility because of its impact on progesterone. While there have been scientific studies to disprove this, yam is still not recommended for women taking OCPs.
- Naturopaths use soy as a treatment for hormonal imbalances during menopause or from conditions like polycystic ovarian syndrome. Soybeans contain natural hormone-like compounds that mimic the role of estrogen in the body. These hormonal effects of soy are believed to interact with OCPs.
- Dairy, specifically milk from dairy farms where cattle is treated with growth hormones like recombinant bovine growth hormone (RBGH) to increase a cow's milk production. Consuming large amounts of RBGH-treated milk could, potentially, interact with OCPs. Milk, however, is an important source of nutrition for women, so chemical and hormone-free, or organic, milk is best.

Medications, however, are more likely to interact with OCPs, or any other hormone type of birth control like the patch, vaginal ring, or injectable, long-acting forms. The types of medications include the following:

1. *Antibiotics.* Most common antibiotics, for example, those that treat upper respiratory tract infections or urinary tract infections, are generally safe and pose no threat to the effectiveness of OCPs. However,

stronger classes of antibiotics, for example, a drug like Rifampin that is used to treat tuberculosis, can weaken the efficacy of OCPs. Since new generations of antibiotics are continually entering the market, it is often safer for a woman to use a backup method of contraception like condoms or abstain from sex while taking a course of antibiotics.

2. *Anti-HIV drugs.* Several of the antiretroviral medications can weaken the efficacy of OCPs and increase the possibility of an unplanned pregnancy. Among these include drugs like darunavir, efavirenz, lopinavir and ritonavir combined, and nevirapine. However, not all HIV drugs interact with OCPs; a woman's health-care practitioner will help her navigate her options.

3. Antifungal medications are believed to potentially weaken the efficacy of OCPs. The use of antifungals is common, especially to treat vaginal yeast infections or athlete's foot. Over-the-counter preparations, however, should be used cautiously. A woman's health-care practitioner can prescribe her an antifungal cream or tablet that is safe to use with OCPs.

4. *Anti-seizure medications.* Several medications that are used to control epilepsy or the onset of seizures can break down the hormones in OCPs. Once this occurs, the OCPs become weak and possibly are not a fully effective form of contraception. Specific anti-seizure medications that break down hormonal OCPs include:

    *   Carbamazepine (e.g., Tegretol, Equetrol, Carbatrol)
    *   Topiramate (e.g., Topimax)
    *   Phenytoin (e.g., Dilantin)
    *   Oxcarbazepine (e.g., Trileptal)
    *   Felbamate (e.g., Felbatol)
    *   Primidone (e.g., Mysoline)

    This list, however, is not exhaustive, and other anti-seizure medications are currently available on the market. Their effect on hormonal birth control, including OCPs, has not been clearly established. Further, anti-seizure medications are intended to be taken daily and often for prolonged periods of time (e.g., months or years). It is advised that women who require anti-seizure medication explore with their health-care practitioner alternative forms of contraception such as diaphragms, condoms, or a nonhormonal intrauterine device instead of using OCPs.

5. *Stimulants.* Drugs used to treat symptoms of specific sleep disorders like sleep apnea or narcolepsy, such as Provigil (modafinil), lessen the effectiveness of OCPs. These stimulant drugs, however, are also used

more commonly to treat symptoms related to attention deficit hyper-activity disorder, jet lag, or to combat the effects of shift work.

6. *Herbal preparations.* Several herbal preparations do not interact well with OCPs. These include the following:

- St. John's Wort—used to treat mild depression or sleep distur-bances, St. John's Wort was demonstrated to contribute to higher rates of breakthrough bleeding and an increased breakdown of estrogen in women who use OCPs and St. John's Wort together. An alternative form of contraception, or a different herbal or prescription medication for other symptoms, should be explored instead of using OCPs and St. John's Wort together.
- Other herbal preparations that have been implicated to weaken the effectiveness of OCPs include saw palmetto, alfalfa, garlic pills, and flaxseed.

Because the scientific evidence related to the exact relationship between herbal preparations and their impact on OCPs is weak or incon-clusive, women should have an open discussion with their health-care practitioner and provide a list of all over-the-counter and prescription medications, and herbal preparations, used and the reasons for taking them. The health-care practitioner can evaluate if an alternative con-traceptive method is warranted or if an alternative medication or supple-ment could be used to allow safe use of OCPs.

38. How does the "morning after" pill work, and how often can I use it?

The "morning after" pill was created because there are multiple instances where birth control, regardless of the method used, can fail. The most common failure is when unprotected sex occurs. A woman is exposed to her partner's semen, and conception, or pregnancy, can occur. It is import-ant to understand how the different birth control methods can fail.

Barrier methods like the male or female condom and the diaphragm are most commonly used. Condoms come in a various sizes and contours, yet many people falsely believe that condoms are "one size fits all." However, poorly fitting condoms can allow seminal fluid or ejaculated semen to leak outside the condom ring. Similarly, a poorly fitting female condom can slip during vigorous sexual activity and allow the penis, seminal fluid, or ejaculated semen to slip inside the vagina between the female condom and the vaginal walls. Diaphragms, while typically well fitted by a health-care practitioner prior to initiation, can also slip if a woman's body changes (e.g., after weight loss or childbirth) or have small holes or tears within the diaphragm itself. Barrier methods can protect against pregnancy only if the barrier method is intact. Therefore, if the barrier method cannot provide full, occlusive coverage against sperm coming in contact with the vagina or cervix, a woman is vulnerable to conception occurring.

The hormonal birth control methods like oral contraceptive pills (OCPs), the vaginal ring or, the hormonal patch are highly reliable forms of birth control. However, these methods work only when used properly and consistently according to a health-care practitioner's instructions or the manufacturer's directions. When a woman misses doses of OCPs and does not catch up with additional doses or does not use a backup method like condoms when indicated, she can be susceptible to conception occurring with sexual activity. Similar risks exist, although less common, with long-term, injectable forms of contraception if follow-up injections are missed or with an intrauterine device if it slips out of place.

Since there can be multiple reasons or circumstances for birth control to fail, the morning after pill, or emergency contraception, was developed to provide women additional protection against becoming pregnant. The most common emergency contraceptive pills contain levonorgestrel, a synthetic form of the hormone progesterone. When taken within 72 hours (or 3 days) of unprotected sex, emergency contraception works to prevent pregnancy by doing one of three things depending on what day of the menstrual cycle the emergency contraceptive pill is taken: (1) may temporarily stop the release of an egg from an ovary, (2) prevent fertilization, or (3) prevent a fertilized egg from attaching to the uterus. The sooner the emergency contraception is taken, the more effective it can be. Emergency contraception can be taken up to five days after unprotected sex and still be effective.

Emergency contraception is readily available at most drug stores and pharmacies. No prescription is needed to obtain the drug. A prescription from a health-care practitioner may be necessary, however, if a woman wants her emergency contraception covered by her insurance plan or carrier. Several brands of emergency contraception are available on the market with varying price ranges, including Plan B One-Step and Take Action by Teva Pharmaceuticals, My Way (Gavis), or After Pill (Syzygy Therapeutics). The dose for most formulations of emergency contraception is similar: one pill taken immediately after purchasing. One dose is usually sufficient, and taking additional or extra doses does not improve the contraceptive ability nor change the likelihood of becoming pregnant. Additional doses could, in fact, cause more unpleasant side effects.

A common side effect of emergency contraception is nausea and vomiting. Taking the emergency contraception with food and not on an empty stomach helps decrease nausea. If vomiting occurs immediately after taking the emergency contraceptive pill, an additional dose may be necessary.

The emergency contraceptive pill, however, is not ideal for every woman. Women who have any of the following should check first with their health-care practitioner (or ask the pharmacist) to determine if emergency contraception is an ideal option:

- Undiagnosed, abnormal vaginal bleeding
- Known or suspected breast cancer
- Active liver disease or a liver tumor
- Diabetes
- Hypertension
- Currently breastfeeding
- Taking any prescription medication

It is important to emphasize that the emergency contraceptive pill is only meant to provide an additional layer of hormonal protection to help prevent pregnancy. It does not cause, or induce, an abortion; if an egg has already been fertilized, emergency contraception has no effect on the fertilized egg. Emergency contraception works to prevent implantation of a fertilized egg by making the uterine lining unfavorable to implantation. However, once fertilization and implantation have occurred, emergency contraception will not be effective.

Because emergency contraception is not an effective form of birth control, women should not rely on it as their go-to method. While a woman may use the emergency contraceptive pill whenever she feels it is needed, she should seek and use a more reliable form of contraception that works with her lifestyle and one that is most likely to be used properly and consistently.

❖

Long-Acting Contraception

39. What is the patch, and how does it work?

Long-acting hormonal, reversible birth control has evolved over the past two decades and now includes the transdermal contraceptive patch or simply "the patch." The transdermal patch (available currently as Xulane in the United States and Evra in Europe and Canada) is a safe, simple, and affordable birth control method that a woman wears on the skin of her upper arm, abdomen, buttocks, or back. The patch is applied, and changed, weekly (i.e., one patch is worn for a week for three consecutive weeks in a month). While in place, the patch delivers hormones gradually and consistently across the skin surface and into the bloodstream to prevent pregnancy. Typically, the patch is removed for one week to allow a monthly menstrual period to occur. Following the menstrual period, a woman can resume using the patch again for the same three-week cycle the next month and each month thereafter.

Mechanism of Action

The patch contains synthetic forms of estrogen and progesterone. The hormones (e.g., norelgestromin and ethinyl estradiol) are in different concentrations compared to other hormonal birth control methods (i.e., the patch typically contains 35 micrograms of estrogen, exposing women to 60 percent more estrogen than the low-dose hormonal contraceptive formulations). The estrogen component of the patch works to prevent pregnancy by suppressing ovulation or stopping the ovaries from releasing an egg. If ovulation does not occur, there is no egg available for a male sperm to fertilize. The progestin component of the patch works to thicken the mucus that surrounds the cervix. Thicker cervical mucus impedes sperm's ability to swim toward an egg if one should happen to be released. The patch, however, offers no protection against sexually transmitted diseases (STDs).

The transdermal patch is a unique method for delivering the hormones into a woman's body. One side of the patch contains the medication (i.e., hormones), which is formulated into the skin contact adhesive. The skin is the largest organ in the body. It covers and protects the body, regenerates when needed, and provides limited, but essential, permeation (i.e., allows substances to pass into and out of the skin layers).

The skin has three layers: the epidermis, dermis, and hypodermis (or subcutaneous). The epidermis is the outermost layer of the skin that contains the stratum corneum. The stratum corneum is the skin's primary barrier against foreign substances entering the body. The patch, then, is adhered to the epidermal layer.

The second layer, the dermis, lies beneath the epidermis and contains connective tissues that give the skin its structure and strength. The dermis also contains hair follicles and sweat glands. The dermis transmits medication from the patch into the deepest layers of the skin.

The third and deepest layer of the skin is the hypodermis. It is the deeper subcutaneous tissue and is made of fat and more connective tissue. This layer also contains blood vessels that also extend back to the dermis and epidermis. As the layers of skin absorb the hormones from the transdermal patch, the hormones are subsequently absorbed via the blood vessels into a woman's bloodstream. From the bloodstream, the hormones are then carried through a woman's circulatory system throughout a woman's body.

Benefits

The transdermal method of delivering hormonal contraception has several benefits over other methods like oral contraceptive pills (OCPs), the long-acting hormonal injection, or contraceptive implants. The transdermal patch is a direct-to-bloodstream delivery system that bypasses the liver's metabolic activity. A woman's body heat activates the patch, prompting it to begin releasing doses of hormones through the skin into the bloodstream.

Second, the hormones supplied are done gradually and constantly as opposed to the large single dose at one time of an OCP. The patch uses the skin's natural barrier properties to achieve a constant permeation of the hormones to achieve steadier blood levels compared to OCPs or the long-acting hormonal injectable.

Third, hormones delivered through the patch bypass the digestive enzymes found in the stomach and gastrointestinal (GI) tract. Traditional pills, including OCPs, enter the GI tract after being taken orally and swallowed and get broken down by the acid in the stomach. The breakdown in the GI tract can diminish some of the hormones' effectiveness. In addition, bypassing the GI tract helps reduce some side effects like nausea.

Finally, the patch is painless and convenient. The patch is simply placed onto the skin, worn for a week, and then removed or replaced. A woman can apply and replace the patch herself at a time that is best for her. The patch is also inexpensive and is typically covered by most insurance plans in the United States.

If used correctly, the patch is 99 percent effective at preventing pregnancy. Proper and consistent use of the patch involves changing the patch on time each week and ensuring the patch is securely adhered to the skin and not peeling or falling off.

Contraindications

While most women will be candidates for using the patch, it is contraindicated in women with the following:

- Benign tumor of the liver or liver cancer
- Breast cancer or a family history of breast cancer
- Uterine cancer
- Estrogen-dependent tumors
- Diabetes
- High cholesterol
- High triglycerides
- Hepatic porphyria
- A history of heart attack (i.e., myocardial infarction), pulmonary embolism, stroke, deep vein thrombosis
- A clotting disorder
- Depression
- Migraines
- Uncontrolled high blood pressure
- A bleeding disorder

- Seizures
- Active smoking in a woman who refuses to quit
- Obesity
- Coronary artery disease
- A current pregnancy diagnosis

Initiation

If a woman is interested in using the patch as a form of long-acting, reversible hormonal birth control, she should consult her health-care practitioner. The health-care practitioner will thoroughly review her medical, surgical, obstetrical, menstrual, and sexual histories and discuss which options are best for her. Both a physical and pelvic examination will occur along with STD screening and a pregnancy test if indicated.

If a woman is a candidate for using the patch, she will receive detailed education about using the patch and a prescription for a box of patches that she can fill at a pharmacy. Typically, the patches are packaged as a one-month supply. Each patch is sealed in a protective foil covering. The patch itself is beige, pink, or flesh colored depending on the manufacturer and square or round shaped. The hormonal medication is contained in the center and, along with the perimeters, contains the strong adhesive that keeps the patch adhered to the skin for a week.

The "first day start" is usually recommended for initiating the patch. A woman will apply her first patch on the first day of her menstrual period. She will not need a backup method like condoms with a first day start. However, a woman may opt to use the "Sunday start" method and begin using the patch on the first Sunday after the start of her period. If a woman uses the Sunday start pattern, she will need to use a backup method like condoms for at least a week to ensure she is adequately protected against pregnancy.

A woman can place the patch on her upper arms, lower abdomen, back, or buttocks. She should avoid using her breasts or areas that are likely to be rubbed (e.g., underneath a bra strap or on inner thighs). The patch should be applied to skin that is clean and dry and not red, irritated, or cut. The skin surface should also be free of lotions, creams, powders, makeup, or body piercings prior to applying the patch. If irritation develops after the patch is applied, it can be peeled off and reapplied to a new area if the adhesive is still strong and adherent.

Once a location for the patch is decided, a woman tears open the protective foil covering and removes the patch from the packaging. Using her fingernail, she gently peels the clear plastic liner off the back of the patch, using caution to not cut, fold, or alter the patch while handling it. The patch is applied with the sticky surface against the skin. Using the palm of her hand or the flat part of her fingers, she will smooth the patch firmly onto the skin, ensuring the edges are secure against her skin without creases or raised gaps. The patch will remain in place for seven days and does not need to be removed for bathing, showering, swimming, or exercise.

Use

A new patch will be replaced on the same day each week for three consecutive weeks. A new patch should be applied to a different area of skin to avoid irritation, or the sites should be rotated every week. The old patch should be folded in half on itself and thrown into the trash and not flushed down a toilet. Any residual adhesive on the skin at the prior application site can be removed with baby oil or lotion. If a woman is late in changing or applying her new patch during the first week of a new cycle, or if she is more than two days late in reapplying her new patch in week 2 or 3, she should apply the patch immediately when she remembers and use a backup method like condoms for one week.

The patch should be checked regularly to ensure it is still in place. If it is partially or completely detached and cannot be reapplied, it should be replaced with a new patch immediately. If a patch has lost its adhesive, a woman should not attempt to readhere it nor use tape or another adhesive to keep it in place. If the patch was partially or completely detached for more than 24 hours, a backup method like condoms should be used for at least a week.

A patch should not be applied during the fourth week to allow a monthly menstrual period to occur. After the fourth week, a new patch can be applied on the same day of the week that the patch was applied in the prior weeks. However, if a woman is opting to skip or stop her monthly period and has discussed doing so with her health-care practitioner, she would continue applying a new patch each week and avoid the patch-free fourth week.

Side Effects

Like other forms of hormonal contraception, there are side effects with the patch. Many women complain about irregular periods, intermittent spotting, or bleeding between periods for the first two to three months after initiating the patch. Other minor side effects include nausea, breast tenderness or swelling, weight gain, acne or pimple breakouts, headaches, mood changes, and irritation, redness, or itching of the skin underneath the patch. However, after three months of consistent use many of the minor side effects should disappear. If they persist past three months of consistent use, a woman should follow up with her health-care practitioner and be reevaluated.

Complications

Like other forms of hormonal contraception, a woman should consult her health-care practitioner immediately if she experiences any of the following signs or symptoms:

- Sharp, sudden chest pain
- Sudden shortness of breath or coughing up blood
- Persistent pain in the calf of the leg or increasing leg swelling
- Sudden, partial or complete blindness or visual changes
- Sudden, severe headaches
- Problems with speech
- Numbness in the arm or leg
- Signs of a stroke
- Yellowing of the skin with fever, fatigue, decreased appetite, dark urine, or light-colored stool
- Severe trouble sleeping or increased feelings of sadness
- A new breast lump that persists through one or two menstrual cycles or increases in size
- Two missed periods or suspected pregnancy

Return to Fertility

A woman can stop using the patch at any time; she simply peels off the current patch she is wearing and does not reapply a new one. Once the patch is removed, she is no longer protected against pregnancy. Furthermore, using the patch should have no impact on a woman's fertility.

After removing the patch, a woman typically returns to her prior menstrual cycle, including ovulation, within one month. Depending on the amount of time a woman used the patch, it may take three or more cycles for her fertility to fully return. Some women may notice irregular menstrual periods after stopping the use of the patch. Women who are overweight may take longer to return to fertility. Fat cells in adipose tissue absorb and store hormones, especially estrogen that could delay their return to fertility.

40. What is the vaginal ring, and how does it work?

The contraceptive ring (also called the vaginal ring, the birth control ring, the "ring," or, by its popular brand name, the NuvaRing) is a safe, simple, reliable, and affordable form of long-acting, reversible hormonal contraception. The ring is unique because it is the only form of hormonal contraception that a woman wears inside her vagina for an extended time. Unlike other forms of hormonal contraception, the ring needs to be inserted only once a month and remains in place for three weeks prior to removal for one week. The ring itself is a small, soft, flexible circle made of ethylene vinyl acetate copolymers that is also latex free. The ring contains synthetic derivatives of both low-dose estrogen (i.e., 15 micrograms of ethinyl estradiol) and progesterone (i.e., etonogestrel).

Mechanism of Action

Once the ring is inserted into the vagina, the surfaces of the ring are in contact with the upper, lower, and lateral vaginal walls. Like the contraceptive patch, a woman's body heat causes the ring to slowly release its hormones. The hormones then get absorbed by the tissues of the vaginal walls. The layers of the vaginal wall tissues contain blood vessels that carry the absorbed hormones into the circulatory system and throughout a woman's body.

The estrogen and progesterone derivatives in the ring work like other forms of hormonal contraception to prevent pregnancy. Once absorbed through the vaginal tissues, the estrogen component suppresses ovulation, so an egg is less likely to be available for a sperm cell to unite with. The progestin component thickens the mucus that surrounds the cervix to impede sperm's ability to swim toward, and fertilize, an egg. The progestin also makes the endometrium, or inner lining of the uterus, thinner and therefore less likely to allow a fertilized egg to implant in the uterus.

The hormones contained in the ring can exert their contraceptive effect only if the ring is in place and in contact with the vaginal walls. The ring remains in place for three weeks and is then removed for one week to allow a menstrual period to occur. When used properly and consistently, the ring has a failure rate of less than 2 percent (or is more than 95 percent effective).

Benefits

There are several advantages to using the ring. First, the ring is convenient for most women. The ring is inserted once (or twice depending on how a woman is using the ring) a month and then a woman is done. The ring typically stays in place despite a woman's physical or sexual activity, protecting her from pregnancy all day, every day. Sex is not interrupted to apply or find contraception. Further, the ring is not affected by illness, nausea, or vomiting.

Second, the ring provides predictable, regular menstrual periods for women. After the ring has been in place for three weeks, it is removed for one week and a menstrual period occurs. Since the progestin component of the ring thins the endometrium, menstrual periods are often lighter and of shorter duration.

Third, the low doses of both estrogen and progestin can also reduce, or help prevent, several medical or gynecologic conditions for women. These include the following:

- Reduced episodes of acne
- Less cysts in the breasts or ovaries
- Prevention of ectopic pregnancy
- Prevention of endometrial and ovarian cancers
- Prevention of iron-deficiency anemia caused by heavy menstrual periods
- Less premenstrual syndrome and menstrual cramps

There are some disadvantages, however, of using the ring. A woman may not be comfortable inserting the ring into or removing the ring from her vagina. There is also an increased likelihood of spotting or irregular vaginal bleeding during the first few months a woman starts using the ring. Temporary side effects like increased vaginal discharge, headache, nausea and vomiting, breast tenderness, or mood changes can also occur. The ring needs to be changed at a specific time each month to remain effective. Finally, the ring does not provide any protection against sexually transmitted diseases (STDs), including HIV.

Contraindications

The vaginal ring is not suitable for all women. Specifically, the ring may not be ideal for women who

- have a blood clot in a vein or artery (or a history of having a blood clot in a vein or artery);
- have high blood pressure;
- are aged 35 or older;
- are active smokers;
- have a history of migraines;
- have had breast cancer in the past five years;
- have diabetes with complications;
- are overweight;
- have weak vaginal musculature that would prevent them from holding the ring securely in place.

Initiation

If a woman wants to use the ring, she should consult with her health-care practitioner. The health-care practitioner will thoroughly review her medical, surgical, obstetrical, menstrual, and sexual histories and discuss which options are best for her. Both a physical and pelvic examination will occur. In addition, the pelvic examination will allow the health-care practitioner to evaluate the vaginal muscles and tissues to determine if a woman will be able to retain the ring for a 3-week/21-day period. STD screening and a pregnancy test, if indicated, may also occur. The ring requires a prescription, and several rings are often dispensed in a box at one time.

A woman can start using the ring at any time during her menstrual cycle. A woman will be protected against pregnancy immediately if she inserts it on the first day of her period. If a woman starts using the ring at any other time during a menstrual cycle, she will need to use a backup method like condoms for at least seven days to be fully protected against pregnancy.

Use

The ring is packaged in a foil wrapper like a condom. After washing her hands, a woman sits on the toilet, squats, or puts one leg up on a chair to have comfortable access to her vagina. After unwrapping the ring, she lightly squeezes the ring between her thumb and index finger. She gently inserts the tip into her vagina and then slowly pushes the ring inside until it feels comfortable. Once inside, a woman lets go of the ring, and the sides then spring open to come in contact with the vaginal walls. Unlike a diaphragm, the ring does not need to cover the cervix to work. Once inserted, a woman should use her index or middle finger to check that the ring is in place. The ring will not get lost inside the vagina.

A woman removes the ring after it has been in place for 21 days. The ring remains out for seven days to allow a menstrual period to occur (if a woman is skipping or stopping her menstrual period following the recommendations of her health-care practitioner, she would immediately insert a new ring after removing the previous one). A new ring is inserted on the same day the following week and remains in place for another 3 weeks or 21 days.

Once the ring is in place, a woman can have sex, use tampons, bathe, swim, or exercise; her physical mobility or activities are not impeded by having the ring in place. At times a woman may feel the ring inside her vagina, but it should not be painful or uncomfortable. Similarly, a male partner may feel the ring during sex, but it should not be uncomfortable or painful for him either. The ring, further, is not harmful to males if the penis comes in contact with the ring.

The ring should remain securely inside the vagina while it is in use. If a woman has vigorous sexual activity, she should check periodically that the ring is in place. If the ring slips out during sex, and she finds it, a woman can reinsert the same ring immediately. If the ring cannot be found, a woman can immediately reinsert a new ring and continue with her scheduled removal and reinsertion dates. If the ring falls out or it has been out for more than three hours, or a new ring is not available, a woman should use a backup method like condoms until she can resume use of the ring. A woman should also consider her need for emergency contraception depending on the length of time the ring may have been out.

To remove the ring, a woman washes her hands and then gently inserts her index or middle finger into her vagina. She will sweep around her vagina until she feels the outer edge of the ring. With her finger on the outer edge of the ring, she gently guides the ring out of her vagina. The ring should come out whole and be discarded in a bag inside the trash; used rings should not be flushed down a toilet. In addition, removal should be painless. However, if there is pain or bleeding or the ring cannot be found or removed, a woman should call her health-care practitioner.

Side Effects

Side effects related to using the ring are related to the combination of the hormones estrogen and progesterone that are contained within the ring. Therefore, common side effects include the following:

- Vaginal infections or irritation
- Vaginal itching or discharge

- Headache
- Nausea and/or vomiting
- Bloating
- Changes in weight or appetite
- Breast tenderness
- Dizziness
- Fatigue
- Changes in the skin or acne
- Hair growth or hair thinning
- Changes in menstrual periods
- Painful menstrual periods
- Possible changes in sex drive

Complications

Like other forms of hormonal contraception, there are risks of serious complications associated with the use of the ring.

1. *Blood clots.* The combination of estrogen and progesterone in the ring increases the risk of serious blood clots that can lead to a stroke, heart attack, pulmonary embolism, or a deep vein thrombosis in the limbs. These risks are increased in women who are smokers, obese, or more than 35 years.
2. *Toxic shock syndrome (TSS).* TSS is caused by bacteria that can be introduced by any object inserted in the vagina, including the ring. Bacteria can easily enter through the vagina and spread to the uterus, fallopian tubes, abdomen, and any of the internal organs. TSS is a rare but life-threatening condition whose symptoms often mimic the flu initially (e.g., fever, abdominal pain). Other possible symptoms include sudden high fever, body rash like sunburn, especially on the soles of the hands or feet, nausea and vomiting, confusion, and dizziness. A woman should contact her health-care practitioner immediately if any of these symptoms develop.
3. Liver problems and the possibility of developing liver tumors.
4. High blood pressure.
5. Gall bladder problems.

Return to Fertility

The ring is like other forms of hormonal contraception because it does not impair fertility. Thus, there are no lasting negative effects on fertility with the ring. Once a woman removes the ring and does not reinsert it, she becomes unprotected against pregnancy. Following the ring-free week when a menstrual period typically occurs, a woman should resume her previous pattern of ovulation in the following month since she is no longer receiving the combination of hormones from the ring that suppresses ovulation. However, after stopping her use of the ring, a woman may notice irregular periods or spotting during the next one or two cycles. Because of the potential menstrual irregularity, women are often advised by health-care practitioners to wait one or two cycles to pass and regulate before attempting to conceive.

41. What is an IUD, and how does it work?

One of the most popular forms of long-acting, reversible hormonal birth control is the intrauterine device (IUD). The IUD has been used since the 1960s. Original IUDs were made with plastic and were intended to be inserted into the uterus without having to dilate the cervix. Today, the modern IUD is a small device made of soft, flexible polyethylene that is shaped like a "T." Several brands of the IUD are currently available on the market (e.g., Mirena, ParaGard, Kyleena), which contain either synthetic hormones (e.g., levonorgestrel) or copper. A prescription is required to use an IUD, and it requires insertion by a health-care practitioner.

Mechanism of Action

The IUD is inserted directly into the uterus and comes in contact with the uterine walls. The IUD releases either a synthetic form of the hormone progestin (i.e., levonorgestrel) or copper into the uterus depending on the type of IUD used. Both progestin and copper prevent sperm from fertilizing an egg: copper acts as a spermicide, and progestin thickens the cervical mucus to block sperm from reaching an egg. In the unlikely event that an egg does get fertilized and survives, both types of IUD cause local inflammation in the uterus that makes it harder for a fertilized egg to implant. Hormonal IUDs also cause thinning of the uterine lining, further making implantation difficult.

IUDs have an annual failure rate well below 1 percent. This means that the IUD is as effective as surgical sterilization; however, unlike sterilization, an IUD is reversible. Most women become fertile again shortly after an IUD is removed. The length of time an IUD remains in place varies. Copper IUDs can remain in place, and continue to be effective, for up to 10 years. Hormonal IUDs, however, are advertised to be effective to prevent pregnancy for five to seven years.

Most women are candidates to have an IUD inserted, including women who are currently breastfeeding, have recently had a baby, or have never given birth to a baby. Because IUDs exert their contraceptive effects directly on the uterus itself, most do not affect breast milk supply, volume, or composition. Hormonal IUDs, further, are ideal for women with heavy periods or painful monthly menstrual periods because they typically decrease menstrual bleeding and cramps.

Benefits

There are several benefits for women who use the IUD. These include the following:

- The IUD is estrogen free, so more women can use it. The copper IUD is completely hormone free.
- The IUD is more than 99 percent effective at preventing pregnancy.
- There is no way to miss doses or forget to use it.
- There are no devices to insert (e.g., a diaphragm) nor barriers to apply (e.g., condoms or spermicides) prior to use.
- No prescription refills are needed.
- The IUD remains in place, and continues to prevent pregnancy, for several years.
- There is decreased menstrual cramping.
- There is decreased, lighter, or absent, menstrual periods while the IUD is in place.
- The IUD is reversible and can be removed at any time.
- The IUD does not impact a woman's future fertility nor make it harder for her to get pregnant in the future.

Contraindications

The IUD is not appropriate for women with certain medical conditions. These include the following:

- Current or previous pelvic inflammatory disease (PID)
- Known or suspected pregnancy

- Gynecologic bleeding disorders
- History of an ectopic pregnancy
- Suspected cancer of the genital tract
- Uterine abnormalities or tumors that would impede the placement of an IUD

Insertion

If a woman desires an IUD, she should meet with her health-care practitioner to discuss her options for contraception. The health-care practitioner will review her medical, surgical, menstrual, sexual, and obstetrical histories. A pregnancy test is likely to ensure a woman is not currently pregnant immediately prior to the IUD insertion. A pelvic examination is also likely to ensure there are no uterine abnormalities or signs of PID. During the pelvic examination, the health-care practitioner may also test for chlamydia and gonorrhea; the health-care practitioner will likely wait until the tests for chlamydia and gonorrhea are confirmed negative before inserting an IUD.

If a woman is found to be an ideal candidate for an IUD, the device can be inserted at any time, including during or immediately after a menstrual period or after giving birth. An IUD can typically be inserted in a health-care practitioner's office or at a clinic. Similar to a pelvic examination, a woman will fully undress from the waist down and lie on her back on an exam table with her feet in stirrups.

The health-care practitioner will insert a speculum into the vagina and use a light to fully visualize the cervix. The cervix is cleaned with an antiseptic solution. A small instrument is used to grasp the cervix which some women will feel as a short, sharp pinch or pain. With a firm grasp of the cervix, the health-care practitioner can straighten the cervical canal so he or she can measure the depth of the uterine cavity to properly place the IUD. Most IUDs come prepackaged and ready for insertion with an applicator by the manufacturer; the health-care practitioner can easily deploy the IUD inside the uterine cavity using the applicator. Women will likely feel a brief cramping sensation when the IUD is deployed.

Once the IUD is in place, the applicator is removed and the IUD arms spring open into the "T" formation. A woman will not feel the IUD inside her uterus. Two strings are firmly attached to the end of the IUD by the manufacturer that will hang down through the cervix. The health-care practitioner trims the strings at the time of insertion, so only a few inches protrude into the vagina. These strings allow a woman to check regularly that her IUD is in place, and later they allow a health-care practitioner to remove the device.

Some women may feel back pain or cramping for a few days after an IUD in inserted. Ibuprofen or acetaminophen can reliably alleviate the discomfort. A follow-up appointment with the health-care practitioner is recommended, usually within a month or following the next menstrual period, to ensure the IUD is in place and there are no signs of infection. The IUD will be checked at every annual gynecologic examination thereafter while it is in place.

A copper IUD is effective as contraception immediately after insertion. The progestin IUD is effective immediately if it is inserted within seven days after the start of a menstrual period. Otherwise, a woman will need to use a backup form of contraception like condoms for at least one week following the insertion of a progestin IUD. However, it is recommended that a woman continue to use a backup method for one month following the insertion of a copper or progestin IUD because the risk of expulsion of the IUD is highest during the first few weeks following insertion.

Checking Placement

A woman will need to check regularly that her IUD is in place. While most IUDs remain securely in place inside the uterine cavity, an IUD can get pushed through the cervix, or expelled completely, without a woman noticing. Checking an IUD is an easy process that a woman will perform monthly, typically after her menstrual period.

After washing her hands, a woman will either sit on a toilet, squat on the floor, or stand with her leg up on a chair to allow her comfortable access to her vagina. She will put her index or middle finger of either hand into her vagina and feel for her cervix. She should be able to feel two strings coming out of her cervix, like the feel of fishing line. She only needs to confirm the strings are present and should avoid tugging or pulling the strings.

If a woman cannot feel the strings, or if she feels the IUD itself poking through her cervix into the vagina, she should notify her health-care practitioner and use a backup method like condoms or abstinence until the IUD's location can be confirmed. The health-care practitioner will likely perform a pelvic examination to determine the IUD's location. An ultrasound (i.e., sonogram) may also be used to scan for, and confirm, the IUD's location within the uterus. An IUD that is poking through the cervix will be removed and, if desired, a new IUD will be reinserted.

Side Effects

The most common side effect reported with both progestin and copper IUDs is irregular vaginal bleeding or spotting. Women with a progestin IUD report very irregular bleeding or spotting for the first three to six months after the IUD is inserted. Bleeding or spotting, however, becomes lighter over time, and some women with a progestin IUD have extremely light, infrequent, or absent monthly menstrual periods thereafter. Cramping and discomfort with menstrual periods typically diminishes or disappears with a progestin IUD. Copper IUDs cause irregular vaginal bleeding and spotting also. However, with a copper IUD, menstrual periods become heavier and last longer during the first three to six months after insertion and may remain heavy compared to before the copper IUD was inserted. Cramping or discomfort with monthly periods can also persist or be unchanged with a copper IUD.

Other common side effects of both copper and progestin IUDs include skin changes (e.g., acne), breast tenderness, mood changes, nausea, ovarian cysts, or weight gain.

Risks

While the IUD is generally safe for use in most women, there are some risks associated with its use. Women with an IUD are at a higher risk of developing PID, which can lead to scarring or obstruction of the fallopian tubes. This damage to the fallopian tubes can lead to future infertility (women who have never given birth, then, are carefully screened and assessed to ensure an IUD is an ideal choice of contraception prior to having an IUD inserted). In addition, damage or infection in the fallopian tubes associated with IUD use can increase a woman's risk of ectopic pregnancy (i.e., a pregnancy in which the fertilized egg implants outside of the uterus). Another rare risk associated with IUD use is perforation of the uterus, where the IUD punctures, or pops through, the uterine wall. Conversely, an IUD, though typically secure inside the uterine cavity, can be unexpectedly expelled from, or fall out of, the uterus.

Complications

The most serious complication associated with both copper and progestin IUDs is infection, specifically PID. IUDs offer no protection against sexually transmitted diseases. PID is an infection of the female reproductive organs that occurs when sexually transmitted bacteria spread from the vagina to the uterus, fallopian tubes, or ovaries. PID can lead to scarring of the fallopian tubes, which could cause ectopic pregnancy (i.e., a pregnancy that occurs outside of the uterus, typically in the fallopian tube) or fertility issues in the future.

The IUD can also perforate through the uterine wall and lead to infection, pain, or bleeding. Women with a copper or progestin IUD are instructed to immediately contact their health-care practitioner if they observe any of the following warning signs that could signal a possible complication from an IUD:

- Abdominal pain
- Heavy vaginal bleeding
- Abnormal spotting or vaginal bleeding
- Unexplained fever
- Smelly vaginal discharge

Pregnancy, though rare, can also occur. If a woman thinks she may be pregnant with an IUD in place, she should contact her health-care practitioner. Her health-care practitioner will perform a physical examination, pelvic examination, an ultrasound, and most likely laboratory blood tests to determine if a woman is indeed pregnant and if the pregnancy is intrauterine (i.e., implanted inside the uterus) or ectopic. If the pregnancy is intrauterine, a woman can opt to continue the pregnancy and, therefore, need her IUD removed. The IUD can be easily removed by the health-care practitioner if the strings are visible. There is a risk of miscarriage when removing an IUD from a pregnant uterus, but the risk of miscarriage related to an infection the IUD may cause by remaining in place is greater. In addition, if an IUD cannot be easily removed from a pregnant uterus, a pregnant woman will be closely monitored because there is significant risk of preterm delivery if an IUD is left in place during pregnancy.

Removal

When it is time to have an IUD removed, the process mimics insertion. A woman undresses fully from the waist down and lies on her back on an exam table with her feet in stirrups. The health-care practitioner inserts a speculum into the vagina and uses a light to fully visualize the cervix. The cervix is cleaned with antiseptic solution. The cervix is grasped with an instrument to straighten the cervical canal while a smaller clamp is used to firmly grasp the strings that protrude from the cervix. The health-care practitioner gently pulls on the strings and the IUD comes out. The arms of the IUD are flexible and fold easily on themselves as the IUD is pulled through the cervix. However, a woman may feel slight cramping as the device is extracted from the uterus. The removal process, overall, is quick. If a woman is going to continue using an IUD, a new device can be inserted immediately after the old one is removed.

An IUD can be removed at any time during a menstrual cycle. However, if a woman is switching her contraceptive method (e.g., switching from an IUD to oral contraceptive pills), a health-care practitioner may opt to start a woman on the new contraceptive method prior to removing the IUD. This will ensure a woman is completely protected against pregnancy as she transitions from one method to another. A woman can also opt to have her IUD removed if she is ready to conceive and become pregnant.

Return to Fertility

An IUD does not impair fertility because it exerts its contraceptive ability directly on the uterine lining; the IUD does not impact the ovaries or ovulation. Therefore, a woman can attempt to conceive immediately after an IUD is removed. Some women may conceive within their next menstrual cycle, while it may take others four to six months to conceive. Current scientific evidence, however, supports that 85–90 percent of women will conceive within a year of discontinuing the use of the IUD.

42. What is long-acting injectable birth control, and how does it work?

Another option for women who desire long-acting, reversible hormonal birth control is the injectable form of contraception. With the contraceptive injection, a woman receives a dose of hormones injected directly into a muscle site at specific intervals. Because the hormones contained within the injection are formulated in a suspension that breaks down slowly, a woman is protected against pregnancy for several weeks continuously. If a woman is consistent with receiving the subsequent doses of hormones once every 3 months, or every 12 weeks, she will remain protected against pregnancy until she stops using the drug. The injectable form offers convenience because a woman needs only one injection every three months; she does not need to worry about taking pills daily or missing doses of hormones while the medication is active in her body. Further, she does not need to worry about changing or replacing devices like a patch, a ring, or a diaphragm. The medication is directly available in the muscle tissue and remains there until it is completely absorbed over time. Injectable contraception, in addition to being safe and convenient, is 99 percent effective at preventing pregnancy when the administration schedule is consistently followed.

Mechanism of Action

Most forms of injectable contraception contain a derivative of the hormone progesterone (e.g., medroxyprogesterone [MPA]). Common brands of injectable contraception currently available on the market include Depo-Provera (Pfizer, Inc.), Depo-Ralovera (Pfizer Australia, Ltd.), and Sayana Press (Pfizer Ltd., UK). The MPA, however, is suspended in an aqueous solution, making it a long-acting formulation, or depo-medroxyprogesterone (DMPA). The DMPA is injected through a thin needle directly into the muscle of the arms or buttocks. Once injected, the DMPA does not get fully absorbed immediately. Instead, the DMPA is slowly broken down over several weeks within the muscle, thus releasing controlled doses of MPA slowly and steadily into the bloodstream. One dose of DMPA remains active for about 12 weeks, or 3 months, within a woman's body. Prior to the completion of 12 weeks, a woman receives her next injection, and she is further protected against pregnancy for the following 12 weeks or 3 months. If no complications occur, and a woman continues to desire to avoid pregnancy, she can anticipate four injections per year to keep her fully protected against pregnancy.

The DMPA is a form of progestin. Like progestins in other forms of hormonal contraception, the DMPA suppresses ovulation, so an egg is less likely to be available for a sperm cell to unite with. It also thickens the mucus that surrounds the cervix to impede sperm's ability to swim toward, and fertilize, an egg. In addition, the MPA makes the endometrium, or inner lining of the uterus, thinner and therefore less likely to allow a fertilized egg to implant in the uterus.

Benefits

Injectable contraception has several advantages. These include the following:

- Injectable contraception is safe and effective for most women for preventing pregnancy when used consistently.
- Injectable contraception is a viable birth control option for women who cannot use forms of contraception that contain estrogen.

- Most formulations of the injection are inexpensive and covered by most insurance plans.
- Using injectable contraception is discreet; it is undetectable by other people, and no one will know a woman is using it.
- There is decreased premenstrual syndrome.
- There is decreased painful periods (dysmenorrhea).
- There is decreased bleeding during menstrual periods and, therefore, a decreased risk of developing anemia.
- There is decreased risk of uterine cancers.

Disadvantages

There are also some potential disadvantages to using injectable contraception. These include the following:

- Menstrual irregularity, particularly during the first few months of use—spotting or irregular bleeding for several days or longer is common. However, with repeated, ongoing use, the menstrual irregularities decrease and eventually disappear.
- Absence of a menstrual period—for women who rely on the presence of a monthly menstrual period, injectable contraception typically causes amenorrhea, or the absence of a menstrual period. After one year of use, more than 50 percent of women report having no periods, and with ongoing use, the number climbs to more than 70 percent of women reporting no periods.
- Heavy bleeding—in addition to menstrual irregularity or spotting, some women report episodes of unpredictable heavy vaginal bleeding during the first months of use. Although heavy bleeding is not typical, it can be prolonged and inconvenient for women when it occurs.
- Delayed return to fertility is common once a woman opts to stop using injectable contraception (see later).

Contraindications

Most women are suitable candidates for using injectable contraception, especially those between the ages of 18 and 50. Injectable contraception is also a method a woman can use if she is breastfeeding because the DMPA does not alter the quantity, or quality, of breast milk. However, injectable contraception should not be used by women who

- have unusual or irregular vaginal bleeding that has not been fully evaluated by a health-care practitioner;
- may be pregnant;
- have current (or a history of) breast disease or breast cancer;
- have current (or a history of) liver disease;
- have had a previous stroke, heart attack, coronary artery disease, blood clots, or blood clotting disorder;
- are active smokers who are not willing to quit;
- are obese;
- are diabetic;
- have hypertension.

Risks

The use of injectable contraception containing DMPA has been identified through research to cause significant bone density loss in women who used it for long periods of time. The bone loss, although reversible when a woman stops using DMPA, can also be minimized, according to ongoing research, if women using DMPA incorporate regular exercise and a well-balanced diet, especially in younger women. Despite the identified bone density loss, current research supports that there is no appreciable increase in bone fracture risk in women using DMPA.

Initiation

Women who desire injectable contraception will need to contact their health-care practitioner for an evaluation. Injectable contraception is available only by prescription. The health-care practitioner will review a woman's medical, obstetrical, menstrual, and sexual histories to see if she is a candidate for one of the long-acting hormonal methods. The long-acting methods like the injectable contraceptive is ideal for a woman who wants to postpone or avoid the possibility of pregnancy for at least a year or longer. However, like other forms of long-acting contraception, the injectable form does not prevent sexually transmitted diseases (STDs). In addition, this method is ideal for a woman in a monogamous relationship or a woman who is willing to use barrier methods like condoms and access routine STD screening if she has multiple partners.

The first injection is usually given during the first five days of a menstrual period. If the injection is given at any time outside of when a menstrual period is occurring, a pregnancy test may be performed immediately prior to administration to confirm a woman is not currently pregnant.

The injection is performed by a health-care practitioner, including a physician, midwife, nurse, or qualified medical assistant. Like other intramuscular injections, the deltoid muscle in the upper arms or the gluteal muscles in the buttocks are the preferred injection sites. The skin is prepped with an alcohol pad. The injection is typically prepackaged by the manufacturer, and the needle provided is thin yet sturdy to produce minimal discomfort during administration. Like a dart, the injection performed by a skilled practitioner is fast and painless, lasting approximately 10 seconds or less.

Use

If a woman received her dose of DMPA within the first five days of her menstrual period, she is considered protected against pregnancy because the drug begins to work immediately. However, if the drug is administered at any other time during a menstrual cycle, a woman should use a backup method like condoms (or abstain from sexual activity) for the first week after receiving the injection.

A woman is protected from pregnancy for about 12 weeks or 3 months. DMPA can be administered for subsequent doses up to 2 weeks early or 2 weeks late (i.e., 10–14 weeks after the last injection). Most health-care practitioners will schedule the next reinjection by 10½–11 weeks from the date of the previous injection to ensure there are no lapses in the contraceptive protection the injection provides. A woman can anticipate four injections per year. If a woman misses her scheduled reinjection appointment by two weeks, and she has been sexually active, her health-care practitioner may perform a pregnancy test prior to administering her next dose. In addition, a woman who has not had her scheduled follow-up injection can consider using emergency contraception if she has had unprotected sex two weeks, or longer, past her scheduled next dose.

Side Effects

Like other forms of long-acting, reversible hormonal contraception, the side effects of injectable contraception are directly related to the progestin (i.e., DMPA) contained within the preparation. Common side effects include the following:

- Weight gain
- Menstrual cycle changes like spotting, irregular periods, episodes of heavy bleeding, lack of a menstrual period (i.e., amenorrhea)

- Nausea
- Bloating
- Dizziness
- Tiredness
- Drowsiness
- Mood changes
- Breast tenderness
- Acne
- Hair loss
- Rare injection-site reactions like redness, itching, or mild swelling

Complications

Once injected, DMPA cannot be removed, nor is there an antidote to counteract its effects. Like other forms of hormonal contraception, a woman using injectable contraception with DMPA should consult her health-care practitioner immediately if she experiences any of the following signs or symptoms:

- Sharp, sudden chest pain
- Sudden shortness of breath or coughing up blood
- Persistent pain in the calf of the leg or increasing leg swelling
- Sudden, partial or complete blindness or visual changes
- Sudden, severe headaches
- Problems with speech
- Numbness in the arm or leg
- Signs of a stroke
- Yellowing of the skin with fever, fatigue, decreased appetite, dark urine, or light-colored stool
- Severe trouble sleeping or increased feelings of sadness
- A new breast lump that persists through one or two menstrual cycles or increases in size
- Two missed periods or suspected pregnancy

Return to Fertility

Unlike other forms of long-acting, reversible hormonal contraception, return to fertility is slower, often unpredictable, following the use of DMPA. Once injected the progestin MPA is released slowly into the bloodstream. However, MPA is suspended in an aqueous solution that does not, purposely, break down quickly. Therefore, when a woman opts to stop using injectable contraception and desires to become pregnant, the remainder of the DMPA needs to be completely cleared from her system before she will begin to ovulate.

The average length of time for menstrual cycles to return to their prior pattern is typically six months after a woman has her last injection. DMPA is not associated with long-term infertility beyond two years after the last injection. Women who are not ovulating by 22–24 months after their last injection, or who are not pregnant 6–12 months after they resume ovulating, should consult with their health-care practitioner and may require further evaluation from a fertility specialist. Many women (approximately 50 percent) will be pregnant within 10 months after their last injection. It may take up to two years, however, for some women to return to their prior pattern of fertility.

43. What is implantable birth control, and how does it work?

Another safe, effective form of long-acting, reversible birth control is one that is implanted underneath the skin surface and remains in place for a few years. Implantable birth control, or the contraceptive implant, is popular because it is convenient and reliable. Unlike other forms of contraception, a woman using the contraceptive implant does not need to take a pill daily, apply a patch, or worry about a device breaking or slipping. In addition, the modern contraceptive implant is a small, thin device that implants easily and quickly in a woman's upper arm. Once implanted, the device is virtually invisible. Further, the contraceptive implant is relatively inexpensive and typically covered by most insurance plans.

Mechanism of Action

The contraceptive implant is a thin, flexible rod, the size of a matchstick. The implant contains progestin that is released from the implant in small, controlled doses directly into the tissues of the upper arm, which then get absorbed into a woman's body. The small dose of progestin released regularly is sufficient to keep a steady amount of progestin in a woman's body to prevent pregnancy over an extended period (e.g., the most popular current contraceptive implant, Nexplanon, can remain in place for four years). It is 99 percent effective for preventing unwanted pregnancy.

Progestins released from the implant stop the ovaries from releasing an egg, thus halting ovulation. Should an egg be released, the progestin also works to thicken the mucus that surrounds the cervix to stop sperm from traveling to unite with the egg.

Benefits

There are several benefits or advantages to the contraceptive implant. These include the following:

- The implant is estrogen free, so more women can use it.
- The implant is easy to implant with minimal pain or discomfort.
- The implant is discreet and not typically visible once implanted.
- The implant can prevent pregnancy for up to four years.
- There is no chance of missing doses or forgetting to use the implant.
- There is no prescription required, nor is there a device to remember to insert (i.e., the vaginal ring or a diaphragm) prior to any sexual arousal or activity.
- There is decreased menstrual cramping.
- There is lighter menstrual periods or no periods at all.
- The implant is reversible and can be removed at any time.
- There is no impact on future fertility, nor does the implant make it harder for a woman to become pregnant in the future.

Contraindications

The contraceptive implant, however, is not ideal for all women. The presence of certain medical conditions can preclude a woman from being able to have the implant inserted. Specifically, women with any of the following conditions are not candidates for the contraceptive implant:

- Currently pregnant
- Active, or a history of, breast cancer
- History of blood clots (e.g., stroke, pulmonary embolism, heart attack, or deep vein thrombosis)
- High blood pressure
- Coronary artery disease
- Liver disease or cirrhosis
- Smokers who are not willing to cut down or quit

Initiation

If a woman desires long-acting birth control, she should consult with her health-care practitioner. The health-care practitioner will review a woman's medical, obstetrical, menstrual, and sexual histories to see if she is a candidate for one of the long-acting hormonal methods. The long-acting methods like the contraceptive implant are ideal for a woman who wants to postpone or avoid the possibility of pregnancy for at least three to four years and wants the convenience of not having to remember, for example, to take an oral contraceptive pill daily or hormonal injections at regular intervals. Since the contraceptive implant does not prevent sexually transmitted diseases (STDs), this method is also ideal for a woman in a monogamous relationship or a woman who is willing to use barrier methods like condoms and access routine STD screening if she has multiple partners.

Insertion

To obtain a contraceptive implant, a woman will make an appointment with her health-care practitioner. During this visit, the health-care practitioner will thoroughly review her medical, surgical, obstetrical, menstrual, and sexual histories to determine if she is a candidate for long-acting hormonal contraception. The health-care practitioner will also discuss a woman's future fertility plans. If a woman is a candidate for the contraceptive implant, inserting the device is relatively easy.

The insertion site is typically the tissue of the inner upper arm. Once the site is identified, the site is prepped with antiseptic solution to prevent infection. Most contraceptive implants are prepackaged in a kit and ready for fast, easy insertion by the manufacturer. The health-care practitioner will numb the insertion site with a small amount of mild anesthetic injected into several areas of the skin around the insertion site. A small amount of skin around the insertion site is pinched and held firm while the implant is injected with an applicator directly into the tissue. The contraceptive implant deploys quickly and stays secure in its place under the skin immediately. Bleeding from the insertion is minimal. A small bandage covers the insertion site briefly. Other than brief, minimal discomfort from the injection of local anesthetic, the procedure is painless.

If a woman receives the contraceptive implant during the first five days of her period, she should not need to use a backup method like condoms. However, if the contraceptive implant is placed at any other time during a woman's monthly menstrual cycle, it is recommended that she use a backup method like condoms, or abstain from sexual activity, until her next menstrual cycle.

Side Effects

Side effects of contraceptive implants are minimal. The most commonly reported side effects are irregular menstrual bleeding or spotting between periods that often dissipates over time. Other side effects may include weight gain, dizziness, mood changes, or skin changes (e.g., pimples or dryness). More serious side effects like abdominal or chest pain, back pain, persistent headaches, or persistent dizziness should be reported to a health-care practitioner promptly.

Removal

Most women with a contraceptive implant appreciate the convenience it provides them for effective birth control. If a woman desires pregnancy, or needs to have the implant replaced, removal, like insertion, is easy and typically uncomplicated. The original insertion site is prepped with antiseptic solution to prevent infection. A small incision is made in the skin around the implant with a scalpel. The end of the implant is grasped with a small surgical clamp and then the implant is pulled out in one piece. If a new implant is being inserted, it can easily be placed in the prior implant's location or inserted into the opposite arm. Sometimes a single stitch or suture is used to close the incision made for removal. The stitch may be dissolvable or removed in five to seven days. A small bandage is placed over the site temporarily.

Return to Fertility

The presence of the contraceptive implant does not affect or impact a woman's future fertility. The contraceptive implant stops working immediately when it is removed or if the supply of progestin within the implant runs out. Most women return to their prior pattern of ovulation within one month or one to two menstrual cycles. Current scientific evidence supports that 80–85 percent of women will conceive within six months after stopping their use of the contraceptive implant.

44. Are there any noncontraceptive benefits to using hormonal contraception?

Hormonal contraception contains some form of the hormones estrogen and progesterone to prevent pregnancy and control the growth, and later shedding, of the endometrium (i.e., the inner lining of the uterus). Hormonal contraception can also be progestin-only for women who cannot take estrogen; progestin-only hormonal contraceptive products have less adverse side effects than those that are a combination of estrogen and progesterone. As new preparations and formulations of hormonal contraception are developed, additional noncontraceptive benefits from using hormonal contraception have been identified. Women may also be prescribed hormonal contraception not for its ability to prevent pregnancy but for its ability to specifically treat or manage certain medical conditions.

Several noncontraceptive benefits have been identified with the use of hormonal contraception. These include the following.

Reduced Risk of Cancer

Estrogen and progesterone stimulate the development and growth of some cancers (e.g., cancers that have receptors for hormones like estrogen and progesterone, like breast cancer and cervical cancer). Therefore, synthetic versions of those hormones, like those in most hormonal contraceptives, can potentially increase the chance of breast cancer. Similarly, hormonal contraceptives are also suspected to change the susceptibility of cervical cells to persistent infection with high-risk human papillomavirus types, thereby increasing the risk of cervical cancer. However, hormonal contraceptives offer a protective benefit against other cancers.

Hormonal contraceptives suppress endometrial growth and therefore suppress the proliferation of endometrial cells. The number of ovulations a woman experiences in her lifetime is reduced during the time she is actively using hormonal contraception, thus reducing her exposure to naturally occurring female hormones. Finally, hormonal contraceptives lower the levels of bile acids in the blood. The effect of the hormones on the endometrium, ovaries, and bile acids affords protection for women against endometrial, ovarian, and colorectal cancers.

The use of hormonal contraceptives has been found to confer a 50 percent risk reduction for endometrial cancer. Women who used hormonal contraceptives for a longer or prolonged period of years have the greatest risk reduction. Similarly, the risk of ovarian cancer is reduced by hormonal contraceptive use, with the risk decreased by approximately 20 percent for every five years of hormonal contraceptive use. Further, colorectal cancer risk was reduced among women by 18 percent, who were currently using some form of hormonal contraception.

Reduction in Premenstrual Syndrome

Premenstrual syndrome (PMS) is believed to occur when levels of progesterone peak prior to a monthly menstrual period and interfere with the brain's production of serotonin. The changes in serotonin lead to irritability and other mood changes associated with PMS. In addition, the fluctuations in progesterone lead to increasing water retention and the symptoms of monthly water weight gain, swelling, and bloating.

Regular use of hormonal contraception (e.g., the vaginal ring, contraceptive implant, long-acting injectable, combined oral contraceptive pills [OCPs]) helps maintain consistent levels of hormones in a woman's bloodstream, thus avoiding the sudden peaks and dips in hormone levels that exacerbate the symptoms of PMS. Some women who use methods like the vaginal ring or the OCP are advised to skip the hormone-free times with their method (e.g., hormone-free pills in a monthly pack or the week where the vaginal ring is left out) to skip having a monthly period to provide more consistent relief from PMS (or worsening PMS, known as premenstrual dysphoric disorder).

Impact on Ovarian Cysts

During a woman's menstrual cycle, an egg grows in a sac called the follicle inside the ovary. As levels of luteinizing hormone rise in preparation for ovulation, the follicle breaks open and releases an egg. If the follicle does not break open, the fluid inside the follicle can form a cyst. An ovarian cyst is a fluid-filled sac inside the ovary. Often, cysts cause no symptoms but may occasionally cause women to experience lower back or lower abdominal pain and bloating. Most cysts are harmless, but some can continue to enlarge and possibly rupture.

Hormonal contraception (e.g., combined OCPs, the contraceptive patch, injectable or implantable contraception) is used to prevent ovulation. The surges of hormones secreted by a woman's pituitary gland in her brain are suppressed, so ovulation does not occur. Without ovulation, the chance of ovarian cysts forming is reduced. If a cyst is present, symptoms of an ovarian cyst should be relieved. Hormonal contraception does not make any existing ovarian cysts to disappear, but it may prevent new ovarian cysts from forming.

Impacts on Dysmenorrhea and Menorrhagia

"Dysmenorrhea" is the medical term used to describe painful menstrual cramps that occur immediately before or during a woman's monthly menstrual period. Dysmenorrhea can be debilitating for women, and up to 90 percent of women report experiencing painful menstrual cramps monthly. Menstrual cramps are triggered by the release of prostaglandins. Prostaglandins are natural substances that are made by cells of the endometrium and other parts of the body. The prostaglandins made in the uterus cause the uterine muscles to contract and promote shedding of the uterine lining during the monthly menstrual period. If the uterus produces too much prostaglandin, painful menstrual cramps, or dysmenorrhea, occur.

Some forms of hormonal contraception, including combined OCPs, the vaginal ring, the contraceptive implant, the contraceptive patch, and the IUD, contain hormones that work directly on the endometrium. Oral contraceptive pills block the production of prostaglandins, while other forms, due to the progestin formulations they contain, thin the endometrium, thus decreasing the amount of prostaglandin produced. Stopping or skipping menstrual periods also decreases the production of prostaglandin and, therefore, eliminates painful periods.

"Menorrhagia" is the medical term for heavy menstrual bleeding. It is estimated that 10 percent of women will experience heavy menstrual bleeding at some point during their years having periods. Heavy menstrual periods have multiple causes, including uterine fibroids, uterine polyps, obesity, or stress. However, more commonly, the overgrowth of the endometrium each month contributes to heavier menstrual periods.

Hormonal contraception contains some form of a progestin that works directly on the endometrium. Oral contraceptive pills, the IUD, the contraceptive patch, vaginal ring, contraceptive implant, and long-acting contraceptive injection contain hormones that thin the endometrium with each monthly menstrual period. With a thinner endometrium, the amount of shedding is less, hence less menstrual bleeding and blood loss with each period. In addition, some methods allow a woman to skip, or stop, her monthly period, thus eliminating menstrual bleeding completely.

Impact on Fibroids

Uterine fibroids, or leiomyomas, are noncancerous tumors that grow on or around the uterus. Fibroids are categorized by their location among or within the muscle layers of the uterus (e.g., subserosal, intramural, submucosal). While most women may never know they have a fibroid, other women experience frequent symptoms of abdominal or pelvic pain, bloating, and heavy menstrual bleeding. Fibroids are believed to be caused by estrogen and to grow when women are pregnant. They are also thought to slowly enlarge over time as they are exposed to, and fed by, circulating estrogen with each monthly menstrual period.

Hormonal contraception helps block the amount of estrogen secreted by the ovaries each month, thus stopping existing fibroids from enlarging (including formulations with the lowest doses of estrogen). Hormonal contraception helps decrease the amount of prostaglandin produced, which, in turn, helps decrease the painful cramping associated with fibroids. In addition, hormonal contraception helps thin the endometrium, so less menstrual bleeding from the fibroids occurs. It is important to emphasize, however, that hormonal contraception helps control only the symptoms associated with uterine fibroids. Surgery (e.g., myomectomy or hysterectomy), interventional procedures (e.g., uterine artery embolization), and menopause are the only definitive treatment options for fibroids presently.

Impact on Acne

Acne is an inflammation or infection of the sebaceous glands in the skin characterized by pimples, typically on the face. Acne in women is influenced by hormones. When a woman's androgen receptors are particularly sensitive, for example, during different phases of her monthly menstrual cycle, testosterone triggers excess oil (i.e., sebum) production within the sebaceous glands that cause skin cells to become sticky. The sticky skin cells then clog pores and lead to breakouts of pimples. Acne breakouts can be painful; become infected; and cause women anxiety, embarrassment, and social isolation.

First-line treatment for acne involves over-the-counter options like skin cleansers and lotions or other topical treatments. A health-care practitioner or dermatologist may prescribe potent anti-inflammatory, antibiotic, or retinoid medications. In addition, hormonal contraception, especially combined OCPs, may also be a treatment option for women. Hormonal contraception must contain estrogen and progesterone to help stabilize circulating androgens and decrease the production of sebum in a woman's body. Further, hormonal contraception helps block androgen receptors, thus preventing the formation of acne pimples or lessening breakouts. Progestin-only contraceptives (e.g., the vaginal ring, the IUD, contraceptive implant, or long-acting contraceptive injection) have not been demonstrated as effective against acne currently.

Special Considerations

While there are several noncontraceptive benefits to several formulations of hormonal contraception, it is important to emphasize that these medications are primarily intended for contraception. The noncontraceptive benefits are secondary findings discovered from years of data, analysis, and comparison from women using different formulations of hormonal contraception. A woman and her health-care practitioner should discuss the risks and benefits of using hormonal contraception for conditions outside of the need for birth control.

Second, hormonal contraception, regardless of whether it is used as birth control or to treat other medical conditions, carries the same risks and potential harmful side effects. Women who have specific medical conditions that would be contraindicated for using hormonal contraception for birth control would also not be candidates to use hormonal contraception for other medical conditions. A comprehensive assessment and evaluation of risks, benefits, and options by a health-care practitioner needs to occur to ensure the safest, most appropriate treatment option is used.

Sterilization

45. What is a tubal ligation, and how does it work?

Sterilization is a permanent, typically irreversible form of birth control. Once completed, sterilization completely removes the possibility of pregnancy occurring and eliminates the need for birth control pills, shots, or implants that contain hormones, or devices like a contraceptive ring, patch, or diaphragm. For women, the sterilization option available is a surgical procedure called a tubal ligation.

Mechanism of Action

Typical menstrual cycles range from 21 to 35 days, with the average menstrual cycle lasting 28 days. At the beginning of the menstrual cycle, levels of the key female hormone, estrogen, begin to rise. Estrogen is produced in the ovaries, the adrenal glands, and fat tissue. The rise of a stimulating hormone called luteinizing hormone causes estrogen to be produced in those specific areas, thereby increasing the level of estrogen in the bloodstream. As estrogen levels rise, the lining of the uterus responds and begins to grow and thicken. While the uterine lining is growing, one of a woman's ovaries begins to mature an egg, or ovum. By about day 14 or 15 of a typical 28-day menstrual cycle, the egg is released from the ovary, hence the term "ovulation." Women with varying, or unpredictable, menstrual cycles, in contrast, may ovulate before or after day 14. It is within the two to three days prior to ovulation, or the day of ovulation, however, that a woman is most likely to become pregnant.

After the egg leaves the ovary, it travels down the fallopian tube toward the uterus. Hormone levels continue to rise, and the thickened uterine lining is maintained. The surge of hormones changes a woman's natural cervical mucus to become thinner and more slippery to allow sperm to travel easily up into the uterus to meet the egg for fertilization. If a woman has sex during this time, and semen is ejaculated into the vagina, the sperm cells have a convenient path into the uterus to unite with the egg that was released. When the sperm and egg unite, fertilization occurs. The fertilized egg continues traveling down the fallopian tube toward the uterus. The thickened uterine lining is an ideal place for the fertilized egg to embed for nourishment as it continues to develop at a rapid pace.

A tubal ligation purposely breaks the connection the fallopian tube has between the ovary and the uterus. During a minor surgical procedure, the fallopian tube is cut, and the two remaining ends are closed off permanently with specialized surgical clips. The two remaining stumps, or ends, of the fallopian tube are then cauterized, or burned, to further close them off permanently. Because there is a blockage at two different points along each fallopian tube, an egg cannot travel down the fallopian tube; similarly, sperm are blocked from traveling up the fallopian tube and uniting with an egg. Fertilization is prevented from occurring permanently. A woman's menstrual cycle, however, remains unchanged: ovulation continues to occur and the buildup, and eventual shedding, of the uterine lining continues. Menstrual periods continue to occur also. While a sterilization procedure like a tubal ligation permanently protects a woman against the possibility of pregnancy, it offers no protection against sexually transmitted diseases (STDs), including HIV. Barrier methods like condoms will still need to be necessary for women with new or multiple partners for protection against STDs.

Benefits

There are several benefits for women who opt for a tubal ligation. These include the following:

- A tubal ligation is highly effective—because a tubal ligation is permanent, it is one of the most effective forms of birth control (i.e., it is more than 99 percent effective at preventing pregnancy). Once completed, there is no way a woman can make a mistake or compromise her degree of pregnancy prevention. A tubal ligation works 24 hours a day, every day of the year.

- Convenience—after a tubal ligation, a woman in a monogamous relationship has no need for any other form of contraception. While she may still need protection against STDs, there are no prescriptions to refill or products or devices to purchase. A woman can have multiple episodes of unprotected sex and not have to worry about pregnancy.
- No change in a woman's natural hormones—a tubal ligation does not change a woman's normal menstrual cycle, nor does it induce menopause. Ovulation and a monthly period continue to occur naturally. There is also no interference with a woman's natural hormone balance.
- No interference with sexual activity—with a tubal ligation, a woman has no barriers to apply (e.g., condoms or a diaphragm), nor is there a need for her, or the couple, to interrupt progressive foreplay to insert or apply a barrier method. Following a tubal ligation, most women report an improved, more spontaneous sex life.

Disadvantages

Along with several benefits, there are some disadvantages to a tubal ligation. These include the following:

- A tubal ligation is permanent—once performed, a sterilization procedure is intended to be lifelong. While a reversal procedure is possible, it is complicated, expensive, and does not always work (*see* Return to Fertility). A woman should pursue sterilization only if she is certain she never wants to get pregnant again. For women who are uncertain about their future fertility plans, they should consider long-acting, reversible contraception like the intrauterine device, the hormonal contraceptive implant, or the contraceptive injection.
- Sterilization has risks—a tubal ligation is generally safe, but it is still a surgical procedure where risks are inherent. Aside from possible pain and discomfort associated with surgery, there are risks of infection or other postoperative complications (e.g., blood clots) that could compromise a successful recovery.
- Sterilization does not protect against STDs—while a tubal ligation provides a degree of sexual freedom because pregnancy is permanently prevented, sterilization procedures do not protect against STDs, including HIV. A woman will continue to need to use barrier methods like condoms, and participate in regular STD screenings, if she has new or multiple partners.

Contraindications

While most women are candidates for sterilization with a tubal ligation, sterilization is contraindicated in some women. Sterilization is contraindicated in women who

- are allergic to any of the materials used in the operating room or during the operative procedure;
- are allergic to contrast medium or dye;
- are uncertain or indecisive about their desire for permanent sterilization and an end to fertility;
- are pregnant or suspected of being pregnant;
- have uterine anomalies that make reaching the fallopian tube difficult.

Procedure

If a woman desires permanent sterilization, she has two options: (1) have a scheduled surgical sterilization procedure or (2) have the sterilization procedure performed at the time of childbirth. The pathway to access sterilization, however, is similar in both scenarios.

A woman needs to contact her health-care practitioner and schedule an appointment for an evaluation. During the consult, her health-care practitioner will discuss her options for contraception and help her determine if sterilization is a viable option for her. A thorough review of her medical, surgical, menstrual, and obstetric histories will occur. A pelvic examination is included with the physical examination, so the health-care practitioner can assess the uterine anatomy, the ovaries, and the position and contours of the fallopian tubes, if possible. If a woman is an appropriate candidate for a tubal ligation, she will receive extensive education about the procedure, aftercare, follow-up, and an emphasis about the permanence of sterilization and the end of fertility. Informed consent will be obtained. A woman can revoke her consent at any time up until the time of the procedure. The pathway to complete the tubal ligation, however, differs depending on whether a woman is not pregnant or pregnant.

If a woman is not pregnant, the health-care practitioner will schedule an appointment with a hospital or surgical center for a minor surgical procedure. (Note: some states, or specific clinics, have rules or regulations that define the amount of time a woman may have to wait before having the actual procedure to ensure she has adequate time to ask questions or change her mind if necessary.) A woman will stop eating food or drinking liquids about 8–10 hours prior to the scheduled surgical procedure. On arrival at the hospital or surgical center, a pregnancy test may be performed to confirm a woman is not pregnant immediately before surgery. A woman will fully undress and don hospital clothing. An intravenous line will be inserted. Her health-care practitioner, or surgeon, will review the procedure again, reevaluate the woman's health status to be sure there are no changes since her last physical examination, ensure that any additional questions are answered, and ensure that the consent is properly signed. She will also meet the anesthesiologist, who will control her pain and level of consciousness during and immediately after the procedure. Once in the operating room, a woman will have the skin of her lower abdomen prepped with an antiseptic solution to prevent infection. The anesthesiologist will administer medications to relax her and then have her fall into comfortable sleep; general anesthesia is rarely used.

The surgeon makes two small incisions: one around the navel or belly button and another elsewhere in the abdomen. Local anesthesia is used at each incision site. Small, delicate instruments are introduced through the incisions to allow the surgeon to visualize the uterus and its structures. The surgeon grasps the fallopian tube, cuts it in half, and removes a small portion. He or she then clips the ends of the fallopian tube where the cut was made and uses a cautery, or heat source, to burn the stumps of each end of the cut tubes closed. The surgeon then moves to the other tube and performs the same procedure. Overall, the entire procedure is completed in about 30 minutes to 1 hour. The cut pieces of the fallopian tubes are often sent to a laboratory for a pathologist to confirm that fallopian tubes were, indeed, transected. Small bandages are placed over the two small incision sites, and a woman is taken to a recovery area. The sedating medications administered by the anesthesiologist wear off quickly. Once a woman is fully awake, can tolerate liquids or a light snack, and passes urine, she can be discharged home. She may be given a prescription for antibiotics to take for several days after the procedure. Often she will follow up with her health-care practitioner, or surgeon, within one to two weeks. Sex can resume once a woman feels able to engage in sexual activity. A woman will continue to see her health-care practitioner for annual gynecologic examinations and screenings as indicated.

If a woman is pregnant and opts to have the tubal ligation at the time of delivery, a woman has two options. She may have a Cesarean section and the tubal ligation will be performed at the time of the surgery or have the same minimally invasive surgical procedure shortly after a vaginal delivery is completed and before the uterus shrinks, or involutes, that would make visualizing the fallopian tubes more difficult. Most women who have a vaginal birth, however, will be encouraged to fully recover from their delivery and then schedule their tubal ligation as an outpatient in a hospital or surgical center just before they resume sexual activity. A woman can also use barrier methods if she does resume sexual activity and schedules her sterilization procedure weeks after her recovery from childbirth has been completed.

Having a tubal ligation during a scheduled Cesarean birth is convenient and effective for a woman. A woman would schedule her Cesarean section with her birth facility or hospital. Once the Cesarean section is completed and the baby is delivered, the surgeon has direct access to the uterus and easy visualization of the fallopian tubes. It is easy for the surgeon to grasp each fallopian tube with surgical instruments, cut out the required segment, and permanently occlude both stumps of the fallopian tube. The sterilization procedure during a Cesarean section is performed quickly. The abdominal incision is then closed, and a woman follows a normal course of recovery.

Side Effects

The side effects of a tubal ligation are rare. However, there are some side effects women need to be aware of following a tubal ligation:

- Unplanned ectopic pregnancy—women who have had their tubes tied are more likely to have ectopic, or tubal, pregnancies compared to other women. While both ends of transected fallopian tube are clamped and cauterized to not allow sperm to pass, there is a chance a sperm could pass through, especially in women who have their tubal ligation performed before the age of 30. An egg in the residual portion of a fallopian tube is fertilized and grows inside that section of tube because it cannot pass down to implant within the uterus. Ectopic pregnancies are medical emergencies that require immediate intervention by a health-care practitioner.
- Post tubal ligation syndrome (PTLS)—PTLS is a cluster of symptoms that include heavy or missed periods, hormonal imbalances, and problems that mimic menopause. Women report feeling hot flashes, mood swings, anxiety, depression, sleep disturbances, fatigue, or vagina dryness. While the etiology of the syndrome is not clearly defined, it requires a more detailed evaluation from a health-care practitioner.
- Regret—some women regret that they underwent a permanent sterilization procedure. Younger women who have changes in their life situation are more likely to report or experience regret with their decision to undertake permanent sterilization.

Complications

Complications from permanent sterilization are related to the surgical procedure. These include the following:

- Reactions or side effects to anesthesia
- Bleeding from the incisions in the skin
- Infection at the surgical site
- Damage to the organs in the abdomen
- Incomplete closure of a fallopian tube, which could result in pregnancy
- Ectopic pregnancy

Women are instructed to monitor for the following symptoms after a tubal ligation that can be indicative of a possible postoperative infection. These symptoms include the following:

- Pain that is not relived by pain medication (i.e., over-the-counter or prescription pain medicine)
- Any drainage from the incision sites
- Abnormal bleeding from the incision sites or the vagina
- Redness or swelling at the incision sites
- Fever
- Vomiting or persistent nausea
- Dizziness or fainting

Return to Fertility

A tubal ligation is intended to be permanent. Fertility is ended once a tubal ligation is completed. However, some women seek to reverse their tubal ligation and become fertile again. A tubal ligation can potentially be reversed through an additional surgical procedure. During tubal ligation reversal, the blocked segments of the fallopian tubes are reconnected to attempt to make one continuous fallopian tube again. This may allow an egg to once again move through the tube, and sperm to travel up the tube, so an egg and sperm can unite to allow fertilization to occur.

Tubal ligation surgery that causes the least amount of damage to the fallopian tubes is most likely to be successfully reversed. Tubal ligations with tubal clips or rings, however, are less likely to be successful. Procedures that scar the fallopian tubes, like the Essure procedure, are generally not reversible. Tubal ligation reversal is not for all women. Specifically, women who are older and have a high body mass index, have tubal ligation procedures completed using clips or extensive cautery, or have short fallopian tube stumps or remnants are least likely to have a successful anastomosis, or rejoining, of the fallopian tubes.

There are inherent risks with a tubal ligation reversal procedure. These include the following:

- An inability to get pregnant after completion of the procedure
- Infection
- Bleeding
- Additional scarring of the fallopian tubes
- Injury to nearby organs
- Complications from anesthesia
- Potential for ectopic pregnancy

If a tubal ligation reversal procedure is unsuccessful, a woman who continues to opt for another opportunity for pregnancy can consult a fertility specialist (or reproductive endocrinologist) to explore if in vitro fertilization or other assisted reproductive techniques are appropriate and applicable.

46. What is the Essure coil, and how does it work?

Another option for women considering sterilization is Essure. Essure is an implantable device that is intended to remain in place permanently. Unlike a tubal ligation, Essure does not require surgery. With Essure, a health-care practitioner inserts flexible coils through the vagina and cervix and into the fallopian tubes. Over time (approximately three to six months) scar tissue forms around the coils, which creates a natural barrier that keeps sperm from reaching an egg, thus preventing pregnancy. Because the Essure coils stay in place and the scar tissue that forms around them is permanent, it is considered a form of sterilization.

Now Essure has been the focus of investigation in the United States by the Food and Drug Administration. A growing number of adverse events have been reported related to the use of Essure. Examples of adverse events include persistent pain, perforation of the uterus and/or fallopian tubes, abnormal or irregular vaginal bleeding, allergic reactions, or migration of the device out of the uterus and into the abdomen. The future of Essure in the United States, then, remains uncertain. However, Essure is available in several countries outside the United States.

Mechanism of Action

The Essure device is a flexible metal coil that contains nickel and polyester fibers. The device is inserted by a health-care practitioner through the vagina and cervix and secured into the opening of the fallopian tubes. While the device is anchored in the fallopian tube, the body begins to create scar tissue around it. Over time, the scar tissue hardens and creates a natural barrier within the fallopian tube. Because dense scar tissue forms around the Essure coil, an egg is prevented from traveling down the fallopian tube. Similarly, the scar tissue barrier prevents sperm from traveling up the fallopian tube to unite with an egg. Overall, Essure is 99.3 percent effective at preventing pregnancy.

Benefits

There are several benefits to Essure. These include the following:

- Insertion is done without the need for a surgical procedure.
- No general anesthesia is required.
- It can be completed in a health-care practitioner's office or clinic.
- It is permanent because the device does not get removed.
- Essure is hormone and drug free and does not impact a woman's normal menstrual cycle. Its effect is localized to the area where it is implanted.

Contraindications

Essure is not ideal for all women. Women who would not be candidates for Essure include those who

- are uncertain about ending fertility;
- have an anomaly of the fallopian tube where only one coil could be inserted (i.e., both fallopian tubes need to have an Essure coil implanted for the method to be effective);
- have a tubal ligation that failed in the past;
- are pregnant or suspected of being pregnant;
- have delivered a baby or had an abortion less than six weeks prior to the Essure procedure;
- have an active infection or STD in the upper or lower genital tract;
- have unexplained vaginal bleeding;
- have a known or suspected gynecologic malignancy;
- have a known or suspected allergy to contrast medium or dye;

- are currently undergoing chemotherapy or are taking systemic corticosteroids that may lead to delayed or failed in-tube scar tissue growth that is needed for occlusion;
- are allergic to nickel, titanium, platinum, stainless steel, and polyethylene terephthalate.

Risks

Significant short- and long-term risks have been identified with the use of Essure. Short-term risks include the following:

- Mild to moderate pain associated with the Essure placement procedure
- Cramping, vaginal bleeding, nausea, vomiting, dizziness, lightheadedness, and pelvic or back discomfort immediately following the procedure

Long-term risks associated with Essure include the following:

- Unintended pregnancy
- Persistent abdominal, pelvic, or back pain
- Perforation of the uterus or fallopian tubes
- Essure device migrating out of the fallopian tubes and into the abdominal or pelvic cavity

Procedure

If a woman is considering Essure as a form of permanent sterilization, she will first need to consult with her health-care practitioner. During this visit, the health-care practitioner will thoroughly review a woman's medical, surgical, menstrual, and obstetric histories and discuss what options are available for permanent sterilization. A thorough physical examination will occur along with a pelvic examination to allow the health-care practitioner to rule out any abnormalities with the uterus or the fallopian tubes. STD screening tests may also be indicated. Extensive education will be given regarding permanent sterilization, and informed consent may be obtained. (Note: some states may require a specified waiting period between signing consent and completing the sterilization procedure to allow a woman ample time to ask questions or change her mind.) If a woman is a candidate for Essure, a follow-up appointment will be made for the procedure.

On the day of the procedure, a woman is advised to eat only a light meal. On her arrival at the health-care practitioner's office or clinic, she will undress fully from the waist down. The procedure will be reviewed again by the health-care practitioner. Once informed consent is confirmed, a woman will be assisted to lie on her back on an examination table and her feet secured in stirrups to allow her knees to slightly fall apart. The health-care practitioner will gently insert a speculum into the vagina and inspect for any signs of infection or bleeding. The cervix will be cleaned with an antiseptic solution, and a local anesthetic may be used directly into the cervix. A small clamp may be used to grasp the cervix firmly while it is gently dilated open. Once the cervix is opened, a small camera called a hysteroscope will be passed through the cervix to allow the health-care practitioner to visualize the uterine architecture and the fallopian tubes. Once the fallopian tubes are landmarked, the health-care practitioner will thread the Essure device into the opening of the fallopian tube and gradually deploy the device, or coil, into place. Once the device is in place, the health-care practitioner will repeat the procedure on the opposite fallopian tube. After both devices are in place, the health-care practitioner will withdraw the hysteroscope and speculum, completing the procedure.

A woman may feel some discomfort when the Essure is placed. She may also feel a brief, sharp pain or pinching sensation when the cervix is grasped with a clamp. As the health-care practitioner manipulates the small camera or other instruments inside the uterine cavity, women may experience cramping or pain. Cramping may also continue for a few days after the procedure. Pain or cramping, however, is often relieved with over-the-counter analgesic medications.

Essure is not effective immediately after insertion. It takes at least three months for enough scar tissue to form to successfully block the fallopian tubes. Because the development of scar tissue takes several weeks or a few months, a woman is advised to use alternative forms of birth control.

Three months after insertion of Essure, a woman will need to undergo a hysterosalpingogram (HSG) to confirm if the fallopian tubes are permanently blocked. Typically performed in a hospital radiology department or specialized radiology center, the HSG uses a dye injected through the cervix and into the uterus through a small, thin catheter. An X-ray is taken to produce pictures of the uterus and the fallopian tubes. The HSG will reveal if the Essure coil implants are in the correct position and show if the fallopian tubes are successfully blocked. If the fallopian tubes are sufficiently blocked, a woman will no longer need to use contraception. However, an inconclusive HSG will require a woman to continue to use contraception until a follow-up, or repeat, HSG confirms adequate blockage of the fallopian tubes.

Side Effects

A woman may experience a range of side effects following insertion of the Essure device. Typical side effects include the following:

- Vaginal bleeding caused by the insertion procedure and the required manipulation of the uterus
- Mild to moderate pain or cramping following the procedure
- Temporary menstrual cycle changes (e.g., longer, heavier periods than normal or spotting between periods)
- Pelvic, abdominal, or back pain

Other reported side effects include the following:

- Headache
- Fatigue
- Hair loss
- Mood changes, including depression
- Allergy or hypersensitivity reactions
- Joint or muscle pain
- Muscle weakness

Complications

Complications with Essure can arise during the insertion procedure and then after the device has been in place. Complications during the procedure include the following:

- Device breakage, with broken pieces inside the uterus or fallopian tubes
- Perforation of the fallopian tubes or uterus that can cause bleeding, damage to the uterus, bladder, or bowel, requiring the need for emergency surgery
- Reactions to local anesthetic(s)

Once the Essure device is in place, possible complications include the following:

- Device migration into the abdomen or pelvis
- Chronic pain
- Metal allergy

- Additional surgery to remove the device
- Removal of the fallopian tube or uterus (i.e., hysterectomy)
- Ectopic pregnancy
- Development of autoimmune disorders (e.g., lupus, rheumatoid arthritis, chronic fatigue syndrome)
- Pregnancy

Return to Fertility

Essure is intended to be permanent. However, a woman can have the Essure device removed to attempt to return to fertility or to minimize some of the unpleasant side effects she may be experiencing. Removal of the Essure device requires a surgical procedure. The surgical procedure requires the administration of general anesthesia, so the surgeon can safely create small incisions in the abdomen. A small hole is made in each fallopian tube so that the Essure coil can be removed. The tube is then sutured closed. Alternatively, the surgeon may cut out a portion of the fallopian tube containing the Essure device and then connect the two remaining ends together (i.e., anastomosis), the way a tubal ligation is reversed. The procedure takes about an hour to complete. A woman can expect pain or discomfort in the immediate postoperative period. Also, she will likely take a course of antibiotics for several days and require a follow-up visit with the surgeon within several weeks following the procedure.

The chances of a woman becoming pregnant after Essure removal depend on the integrity of the repaired fallopian tube. Extensive scarring within the fallopian tube, or at the anastomosis, is possible. However, the Essure device does not interfere with any of the hormones that regulate the menstrual cycle, so a woman will continue to ovulate according to her usual cycle. What is impacted by having the Essure device is the transportation of an egg down the fallopian tube. Once the Essure device is removed, a woman is more likely to have an ectopic pregnancy than an intrauterine pregnancy. A woman can become pregnant only if a clear path exists within the fallopian tube for an egg to unite with a sperm and then implant in the uterus. Achieving an intrauterine pregnancy after the Essure device is removed can take several months. If a woman continues to opt for another opportunity for pregnancy, she can consult a fertility specialist (or reproductive endocrinologist) to explore if in vitro fertilization or other assisted reproductive techniques are appropriate and applicable.

47. What is a vasectomy, and how does it work?

Men have an option for permanent sterilization. While most birth control options are targeted toward women, the vasectomy is the only permanent sterilization procedure for men. With a vasectomy, a key conduit that permits sperm cells to mix with semen and be ejaculated during a male orgasm is permanently severed. After a vasectomy, a man continues to produce sperm and enjoy sexual intimacy, but his sperm will be absent from his semen and seminal fluid. Without sperm in the semen or seminal fluid, a man's ability to fertilize an egg is impeded.

Mechanism of Action

Sperm is the male reproductive cell that develops in the testicles. Once sperm is produced, it is stored in a structure called the epididymis. During sexual arousal and activity, the prostate gland begins to secrete prostate fluid, a main component of semen, and the seminal fluid that transports sperm cells. Seminal fluid also nourishes the sperm cells and helps keep the sperm motile as they travel toward an egg for fertilization.

As sexual arousal or activity increases, sperm cells in the epididymis join with the seminal fluid and semen made by the prostate. When the male orgasm occurs, the prostate gland helps to forcefully expel the semen and seminal fluid into two ejaculatory ducts called the vas deferens and the seminal vesicles. The vas deferens empties directly into the urethra. As orgasm is completed, semen and seminal fluid is then ejaculated out of the urethra through the opening in the penis.

A vasectomy is a surgical procedure that blocks or cuts each vas deferens tube. If the vas deferens is blocked or cut, sperm cannot be mixed with semen or seminal fluid, thereby making the male ejaculation free of the sperm cells needed for fertilization to occur. Since the sperm does not enter the semen or seminal fluid, it remains in the testicles and gets reabsorbed by the body. A vasectomy is 99 percent effective at preventing pregnancy. However, like other forms of permanent sterilization for women, a vasectomy provides lifelong protection only against the possibility of pregnancy; it does not protect a man from contracting, or transmitting, sexually transmitted diseases (STDs) or HIV.

Benefits

There are several benefits for men to undergo a vasectomy. These include the following:

- Vasectomies are highly effective—since a vasectomy is a permanent form of sterilization, it is more than 99 percent effective. Once completed, a vasectomy prevents pregnancy 24 hours each day, 7 days per week, for the rest of a man's life.
- Convenience—after a vasectomy, a man or couple does not have to worry about a birth control regimen or using a barrier method like condoms to prevent pregnancy. However, for a man with new or multiple partners, the use of barrier methods like condoms and routine STD screenings are needed to prevent contracting or transmitting STDs.
- Improved sex life—a vasectomy allows sexual activity to be more spontaneous or to avoid stopping progressive foreplay or vigorous sexual activity to apply, or reapply, condoms or spermicide.
- No impact on a man's natural hormonal balance—a vasectomy does not interfere with a man's sperm production, virility, or sex drive. He will continue to make sperm because his levels of testosterone are not impacted by a vasectomy. Further, the amount, texture, or appearance of ejaculated semen is unchanged.

Contraindications

Most men are candidates for a vasectomy. However, some contraindications exist, including the following:

- Bleeding disorder that would impede healing after the vasectomy procedure
- Known or suspected malignancy of the testes
- Active or suspected STD(s)

Careful screening by a health-care practitioner will also occur for men who have never had children, are younger than 30 years, or have a severe or chronic illness (e.g., cancer) to determine if a vasectomy is an appropriate option for birth control.

Risks

There are also risks involved with a vasectomy procedure. Immediately after the procedure, men may experience the following:

- Swelling at the incision site
- Bruising to the penis or scrotum

- Bleeding inside the scrotum
- Blood in the semen
- Infection

Long-term risks, though rare, include the following:

- Fluid buildup in the testicle (i.e., hydrocele).
- Chronic pain.
- Pregnancy—despite surgical precision or expertise, there is a remote chance that the procedure will not work. It can also take time for the semen or seminal fluid to be completely free of any sperm cells.

Current scientific evidence has demonstrated that having a vasectomy performed does not impact a man's risk of developing prostate or testicular cancer or erectile dysfunction. Further, no association has been established between men who have a vasectomy and the onset of development of diabetes, dementia, or early onset Alzheimer's disease.

Procedure

If a man desires a vasectomy for permanent sterilization, he should contact his health-care practitioner. The health-care practitioner will thoroughly review a man's medical, surgical, and sexual histories and discuss the man's, or couple's, future fertility plans. A physical examination may be performed, including examination of the penis, scrotum, and prostate to rule out any abnormalities. If a man is a suitable candidate for a vasectomy, he will likely be referred to a physician who specializes in performing the vasectomy procedure (e.g., urologist, urologic surgeon, or urology clinic).

A man will typically need to meet with whomever will be performing the vasectomy prior to the actual procedure. The health-care practitioner performing the vasectomy will discuss the procedure, including its risks and benefits, and provide an opportunity for the man, or the couple, to ask questions. Another focused physical examination of the genitalia is likely. Informed consent may be obtained.

The procedure is typically performed in a health-care practitioner's office or in a clinic. On the day of the procedure, a man may be allowed to eat a light meal and will typically shower with an antiseptic soap. On arrival for the procedure, a man will have his history reviewed and updated and his informed consent verified. A man will undress from the waist down, and a surgical drape will be used to cover the legs and lower abdomen.

Local anesthesia is injected with a small needle into the scrotum. The surgeon kneads the scrotum until he palpates and landmarks the vas deferens. Although there are several variations on the surgical procedure, two small incisions are made in the scrotum, and the vas deferens is pulled closer to the skin surface. The vas deferens is transected, or cut, and the two remaining ends of the tube are permanently sealed. The procedure is done on both the right and left vas deferens. Once completed, the incisions in the scrotum are closed and a small dressing applied. Following the procedure, a man may return home and work but is advised to avoid sex and strenuous sexual activity for at least one week.

A vasectomy is not immediately effective. Existing sperm need to clear out of a man's semen before it is safe for him to have unprotected sex. It can take up to three months for sperm to be completely absent from the semen or seminal fluid. Therefore, sex occurring after the vasectomy procedure will require the use of a barrier method like a condom or diaphragm to prevent pregnancy for several weeks after the vasectomy procedure.

A semen analysis is used to determine if sperm are present in the semen or seminal fluid. At a follow-up visit with the health-care practitioner or surgeon who performed the vasectomy, a man will be asked to masturbate and provide a semen sample for analysis. If sperm is not detectable in the sample, it is likely safe for a man to begin having unprotected sex. An at-home test kit is also currently available.

Side Effects

There are minimal side effects associated with a vasectomy. Typical side effects, however, include the following:

- Pain or mild discomfort that is typically relieved by over-the-counter analgesics, ice, or proper-fitting underwear or support.
- Bleeding or swelling at the incision.
- Bruising of the penis or scrotum.
- Bleeding or blood clots (i.e., hematoma) inside the scrotum.
- Inflammation of the epididymis (i.e., epididymitis) that may require antibiotics.

- Formation of sperm granulomas—sperm granulomas are small lumps that form when sperm leaks from the vas deferens into the surrounding tissue after surgery. Sperm granulomas can be painful but typically resolve after treatment with rest and over-the-counter analgesics.
- Unplanned pregnancy—this occurs typically when men do not adhere to the post vasectomy instructions and have unprotected sex too quickly after the vasectomy procedure or before sterility was confirmed.

Complications

Long-term complications can occur with a vasectomy. Although uncommon, they include the following:

- Post vasectomy pain syndrome—due to nerve damage from the vasectomy procedure that leads to persistent testicular or scrotal pain; also called congestive epididymitis or chronic post vasectomy testicular pain.
- Autoimmune issues—a man's body is not accustomed to sperm cells freely floating in his bloodstream. A vasectomy ruptures the barrier of tissue that blocks sperm cells from entering his bloodstream. As a result, antisperm antibodies form. Although generally harmless, headaches, lymph node enlargement, or adrenal gland malfunction could occur because of the antisperm antibodies.
- Formation of a spermatocele—a spermatocele is an abnormal cyst that develops in the small, coiled tube located on the upper testicle that collects and transports sperm.

Return to Fertility

A vasectomy is intended to be permanent sterilization for a man. However, circumstances in a man's, or couple's, life can change that would steer him to explore having his vasectomy reversed so he can father more children. A vasectomy reversal is possible to undo a vasectomy. Like the original vasectomy procedure, incisions are made in the scrotum and the two ends of the cut vas deferens are located. The two ends are reconnected (i.e., anastomosis) and, once healed, sperm has a conduit to mix with semen or seminal fluid. Success rates with vasectomy reversal vary from 40 to 90 percent. Whether a reversal is successful depends on many factors, including time since the vasectomy was initially performed (i.e., the longer it has been since the initial vasectomy, the less likely a reversal procedure is to be successful), the age of the female partner trying to conceive, or the expertise and skill of the surgeon performing the reversal procedure. Like the original vasectomy procedure, the risk of bleeding, pain, or infection exists with the reversal procedure. Most men will need to refrain from sex or sexual activity for at least two to three weeks after the reversal procedure.

A man, or couple, wishing to achieve pregnancy following a vasectomy may also consider assisted reproductive techniques. If a vasectomy reversal procedure is unsuccessful, a man, or couple, who continues to opt for another opportunity for pregnancy can consult a fertility specialist (or reproductive endocrinologist) to explore if in vitro fertilization or other assisted reproductive techniques are appropriate and applicable.

Case Studies

Case Study 1: Kelly

Kelly is a 17-year-old high school senior. From her freshman through junior years in high school, Kelly was an honors student, active in seasonal sports, and involved with different school clubs. Through her various school activities, Kelly developed a large circle of male and female friends. Before entering senior year, Kelly worked a summer job as a lifeguard at her town pool and met Tom, another lifeguard. Their relationship grew, and by the end of the summer Kelly and Tom were having sex regularly. Each time they had sex they used condoms to prevent pregnancy. However, both Kelly and Tom worried that they might forget to use condoms or have a condom break during sex. Neither Kelly nor Tom wanted pregnancy to occur. During her annual gynecology appointment, Kelly decided to ask the doctor if oral contraceptive pills (OCPs) were right for her.

The doctor reviewed Kelly's medical, surgical, menstrual, and sexual histories. The doctor appreciated that Kelly ate a healthy diet, that she was physically active and exercised regularly, that her weight was appropriate for her age and height, and that she never smoked. Kelly also had regular menstrual cycles every 28 days, with periods that lasted only two to three days. The doctor discussed the various birth control options available to Kelly. Because Kelly, and her family's, medical history was free of cancers, breast disease, blood clots, or liver problems, and Kelly's physical examination revealed that she was currently in excellent health, the doctor agreed that Kelly was an ideal candidate for OCPs.

Along with a thorough physical examination, the doctor performed a pelvic examination. During the pelvic exam, the doctor took a swab from Kelly's cervix to screen her for sexually transmitted diseases (STDs). The doctor also gently palpated Kelly's cervix, uterus, and ovaries to identify the presence of any abnormalities. After the exam was completed, Kelly dressed and sat with the doctor to learn about using OCPs.

The doctor gave Kelly starter packs of OCPs that contained the lowest possible doses of estrogen and progesterone. Kelly was instructed to start her pills on the Sunday following the start of her next period and to take one pill each day, preferably at the same time so she would develop a pill-taking routine and not miss a dose. The doctor reviewed what Kelly should do if she missed pills and recommended she continue to use condoms for the next several weeks until the OCPs were fully effective. The doctor also stressed the warning signs Kelly needed to monitor for like chest pain, headaches, abdominal pain, swelling to her legs, or difficulty breathing. Because the doctor discussed a large amount of important information, she provided Kelly with printed material to review and useful websites to explore so Kelly could be well informed about using OCPs.

Kelly used the OCPs for three months and returned to see the doctor as scheduled. The doctor reviewed Kelly's use of the OCPs and inquired if Kelly was experiencing side effects. Kelly reported that she had some irregular spotting one month after starting the OCPs but that her periods had become shorter and lighter since starting on OCPs. She also reported less cramping during her period that allowed Kelly to continue to play sports. Because Kelly was using the OCPs properly and having minimal side effects, the doctor continued Kelly on her current OCP prescription. Before leaving, the doctor reviewed the prior education she gave Kelly and provided her with additional information on emergency contraception and STD screening. The doctor reminded Kelly to call her if any problems or concerns developed. The doctor also scheduled Kelly's annual exam for the following year, so it would be completed before Kelly left for college.

Analysis

Like many young women, Kelly began to be sexually active without any prior planning. Condoms become the easiest, most inexpensive method of birth control for a couple to use. However, Kelly realized that condoms were useful only if they were used properly and consistently each time she had sex; a more reliable method would minimize the risk of her forgetting to use a condom or of the condom breaking.

OCPs are common, and many women are familiar with their use. However, OCPs carry significant risks, so they are not ideal for every woman. The doctor was careful to assess Kelly for the presence of any risk factors that would preclude her from using OCPs (e.g., heart disease, blood clots, active cancers, liver disease) and reviewed her family's history also. Once the doctor was satisfied that Kelly was an ideal candidate to use OCPs, she chose the lowest dose possible that would give Kelly the protection she needed to prevent pregnancy but also minimize some of the potential harmful side effects of the OCPs. Given that Kelly was still a teenager, it is likely that she would be using OCPs for several years, so providing contraception with the lowest amount of synthetic estrogen and progesterone would aid in protecting Kelly from future complications.

Kelly also began using her OCPs in excellent physical health. Eating healthy, maintaining an ideal body weight with regular physical exercise, and being a nonsmoker are ways Kelly can help avoid some of the problems or side effects that arise from using OCPs. Fortunately, Kelly experienced only some irregular spotting after initiating the use of OCPs and then noticed that her periods were shorter and lighter, typical side effects women can anticipate once beginning an OCP regimen. The doctor, however, took additional time to consistently review potential warning signs, or danger signs, with Kelly at each visit (e.g., chest pain, headaches, difficulty breathing, leg swelling, abdominal pain). Since there is a lot of important information to relay to patients who start, and continue to use, OCPs, the doctor was proactive in providing Kelly with printed material she could refer to along with high-quality, evidence-based websites run by reputable organizations or health-care leaders who could also provide Kelly with any additional information she may need. Further, the doctor realized that Kelly would be heading to college the following summer, so she ensured Kelly had her follow-up appointment for an annual exam and an opportunity to address any birth control needs, or continue her current regimen, before leaving for college.

Case Study 2: Mindy

Mindy is a 30-year-old married mother of four, who works full-time. Following the birth of her last baby, Mindy and her husband decided that four children made their family complete and desired no more children. Mindy and her gynecologist discussed her contraceptive options. Since Mindy had regular, but heavy, periods, she chose the intrauterine device (IUD) because it was safe, was convenient, and could potentially lessen, or stop, her monthly periods.

Mindy appreciated having the IUD in place. Her periods became lighter, she and her husband could enjoy sex spontaneously, and she found it easy to check the IUD strings monthly after her period. However, one day Mindy developed a sudden fever, chills, and abdominal pain. She was also persistently nauseous, she had no appetite, and she could not tolerate any liquids orally. She had generalized body aches, fatigue, and a persistent headache. Believing she had the flu, Mindy contacted her health-care practitioner; on hearing her symptoms, her health-care practitioner sent her immediately to the emergency department of her local hospital for an evaluation.

On arrival at the emergency department, Mindy felt worse. Her fever was over 103°F; her abdominal pain was worsening; and the body aches, chills, and headache were unrelenting. The emergency department physician examined Mindy and discovered she had diffuse abdominal tenderness, some irregular vaginal bleeding, and abnormal, foul-smelling vaginal discharge. Realizing Mindy had an IUD in place, the emergency department physician took cultures from her cervix, ordered laboratory blood tests, and diagnosed Mindy presumptively with pelvic inflammatory disease (PID). An intravenous (IV) line was inserted to give Mindy fluids, and antibiotics were administered. Medications to reduce her fever and control her pain were also provided. Mindy was admitted to the hospital for treatment and monitoring of her symptoms.

The antibiotic regimen, and other medications, improved Mindy's symptoms. The cultures and laboratory blood tests confirmed the diagnosis of PID. Mindy's gynecologist was consulted, and he explained that the IUD can transmit harmful bacteria or other pathogens into the uterus and cause an infection of the uterus, fallopian tubes, or ovaries. Her gynecologist recommended having the IUD removed.

After Mindy was discharged from the hospital and completed a full course of antibiotic therapy, she made an appointment with her gynecologist to remove her IUD. Mindy undressed and was assisted onto an exam table with her feet in stirrups. The gynecologist inserted a speculum so he could visualize the cervix. Using a small clamp, the gynecologist gently grasped Mindy's cervix to hold it firmly in place while he used a second clamp to grasp the IUD strings. With light traction, the gynecologist was able to pull the IUD out of the uterus and through the cervix. During the procedure, Mindy experienced only slight cramping that quickly resolved.

When the IUD removal procedure was completed, Mindy dressed and spoke with her gynecologist. He advised her about her need for contraception and to use barrier methods like condoms until she decided on another birth control option. The gynecologist reviewed PID again and emphasized the signs and symptoms Mindy should monitor for in the future. The gynecologist also suggested screening Mindy's husband for STDs prior to their next episode of sexual activity to ensure Mindy did not get reinfected with harmful bacteria or pathogens.

Analysis

For women like Mindy, the IUD is a convenient, reliable, and safe form of long-acting birth control. The IUD is ideal for women who either finished having children or want to postpone having any additional children for several years. Because the IUD offers no protection against STDs, it is well suited for women, and their partners, who are in an equally monogamous relationship. The IUD affords a couple more freedom for a spontaneous sex life without the potential misuse or failure of other common birth control methods. In addition, the IUD works locally on the uterine lining itself, so it is an ideal choice of hormonal contraception for women who cannot tolerate, or take, other forms of hormonal contraception containing estrogen. While periods initially may be heavy or irregular for the first few months after having an IUD inserted, they typically become shorter and lighter or stop completely once an IUD has been in place for several months.

Most women will have an IUD inserted for several years without complications. There is no maintenance for an IUD other than to check regularly that the strings are still present by feeling for them at the cervix. However, the IUD can have serious complications that need to be addressed immediately. The signs and symptoms of an infection can mimic other conditions. Mindy's symptoms were like the onset of the flu or some other kind of infection. What made Mindy's symptoms more suspicious was the extremely high fever, irregular vaginal bleeding, and the foul-smelling vaginal discharge that would signal a health-care practitioner to rule out causes related to the IUD or within the genital tract. The IUD strings serve as a direct conduit for harmful pathogens to enter directly into the uterus and infect the structures of the genital tract like the fallopian tubes or ovaries. If left untreated, PID can have serious consequences, and a woman can get progressively worse in a short period of time, hence the reason aggressive treatment, with antibiotics, IV fluids, other medications, and hospital admission, was implemented swiftly in the emergency department.

Once Mindy's condition was stabilized and her infection was treated, it was logical to remove her IUD and offer her other options. PID is typically caused by gonorrhea or chlamydia within the genital tract, and most often the pathogens that cause PID are transmitted from one infected partner to another during sex. Mindy's health-care practitioner focused his attention on Mindy's husband and strongly encouraged him to undergo STD screening and possible treatment. Despite treatment, Mindy could still be at risk for contracting PID again if her partner continued to transmit the harmful pathogens to her. If left inserted, the IUD would continue to serve as an easy conduit for those harmful pathogens to reenter the uterus. Removal of the IUD is a simple, minimally uncomfortable procedure that can be completed quickly during an office visit. However, with the IUD out, Mindy was at risk to become pregnant with her next episodes of sexual activity, so a backup or alternative method needed to be agreed upon and implemented prior to her leaving her health-care practitioner's office.

Case Study 3: Mary

Mary is a 21-year-old college student, who lives in a co-ed dormitory on campus. Mary has a steady boyfriend and has been having frequent sex with him for the past two years. Mary and her boyfriend use condoms as their sole form of birth control.

Over a long holiday weekend, Mary and her boyfriend were spending the evening together and had sex. After Mary's boyfriend reached orgasm, he pulled his penis out of Mary's vagina and noticed the condom he was wearing had a large tear along its side. Mary began to panic because she believed she was in the fertile phase of her cycle. Because it was evening time and a holiday weekend, the student health center was closed. Mary's boyfriend drove her to a retail pharmacy where Mary was able to speak with a pharmacist. The pharmacist recommended several brands of emergency contraception that could be purchased over the counter without a prescription. Mary chose Plan B.

The pharmacist instructed Mary to take the one-pill dose of Plan B immediately with food. He cautioned her that she might experience nausea, vomiting, or a headache after taking the pill. He reassured her that if she did experience vomiting, she could repeat the dose of medication.

The pharmacist also advised Mary that there was information about Plan B on the drug's web page and suggested Mary follow up with her gynecologist, nurse practitioner, midwife, or the student health center to explore other options for birth control.

Mary took her dose of Plan B with food. A few hours later she felt brief waves of nausea and a slight headache. Once the weekend was over, Mary scheduled an appointment with the nurse practitioner (NP) in the student health center. The NP commended Mary on acting quickly to access emergency contraception because the sooner it is taken, the more effective it is, but that the drug is effective up to 72 hours after unprotected sex. The NP further advised Mary to monitor for the onset of her next period and warned her that it might arrive sooner or be irregular or heavier than her previous periods. If no period occurred, Mary was instructed to return to the student health center for a pregnancy test.

The NP reminded Mary that emergency contraception is useful only for emergencies and that a regular, reliable form of birth control is recommended for women. The NP then discussed the various birth control options available and appropriate for Mary and gave her additional printed material and websites she could review for more information. Mary took the information and agreed to see the NP again after her next period arrives for a complete physical and to select, and initiate, a new birth control method.

Analysis

Birth control failure can occur with any of the available methods. When a condom used as a barrier method breaks, semen or seminal fluid comes in contact with the vagina or any of the vaginal surfaces and creates an opportunity for sperm to potentially unite with an egg for fertilization. No birth control method, however, is currently capable of destroying sperm cells or an egg. Therefore, the only way to prevent fertilization is to make it difficult for sperm to easily travel toward an egg or, if fertilization has occurred already, to make the intrauterine lining unfavorable to implantation. Emergency contraception typically contains forms or derivatives of the hormone progesterone. Progesterone causes thickening of the cervical mucus, which impedes sperm's travel toward an egg and thins the endometrial, or inner, lining of the uterus so implantation cannot occur.

Mary acted quickly after she and her boyfriend discovered the condom they were using had broken. The pharmacist directed her to several brands of emergency contraception that are typically available over the counter without a prescription. The different brands or varieties of emergency contraception are one or two pills taken within 72 hours of unprotected sex. The pill begins to work within a short period of time. Mary experienced nausea, the most frequent side effect reported with emergency contraception use. Vomiting may also occur, and Mary was instructed that she could possibly repeat her dose of emergency contraception if necessary. However, Mary was advised the common gastrointestinal side effects could be minimized if the emergency contraception pill was taken with food.

When used properly, emergency contraception is highly effective at preventing pregnancy. Women like Mary who use emergency contraception can anticipate some menstrual irregularity and will need to monitor for the onset or arrival of the next month's menstrual period. Pregnancy can still occur despite the use of emergency contraception, so prompt testing may be indicated if a woman misses her next menstrual period. While condoms are a reliable form of birth control if used properly and consistently, there is still a risk of breakage despite careful use. Like Mary, women may explore different options for contraception that best suit their lifestyle and needs.

Case Study 4: Greg

Greg is a 36-year-old man who has three children, aged 10, 8, and 5. After the birth of his last child, Greg and his wife decided that their family was complete, and they were done having children. Because Greg's wife had several medical issues that precluded her from being a candidate for using hormonal contraception or undergoing permanent sterilization, Greg opted to undergo permanent sterilization and have a vasectomy. The vasectomy was completed without complications, and a follow-up sperm analysis three months later confirmed the absence of sperm in Greg's semen.

Three years ago, however, Greg and his wife began having marital difficulties that led them to divorce. After his divorce, Greg began to date, fell in love, and married a 30-year-old woman who had never had children. Following his remarriage, Greg and his new wife decided to expand their family and have more children. Greg needed to explore having his vasectomy reversed.

Greg made an appointment with the same urologist who had performed his original vasectomy. The urologist reviewed Greg's medical history and performed a brief physical examination to assess Greg's penis, scrotum, testes, and prostate. While Greg was a candidate to attempt a vasectomy reversal, the urologist warned him that a return to fertility was not guaranteed. The risks and benefits of the reversal procedure were discussed.

Greg returned to the urologist's office for his scheduled vasectomy reversal procedure. The urologist reviewed the procedure, answered any additional questions, and obtained informed consent. Greg undressed from the waist down, and the skin around his penis and scrotum was prepped with antiseptic solution. The urologist made two small incisions in Greg's scrotum and located the two ends of each severed vas deferens. The urologist reunited the two ends of the tubes and then closed the incision in the scrotum with small sutures. After Greg dressed, he was given instructions about activity, wound care, scrotal support, and using over-the-counter analgesics for pain. Greg was further advised to avoid strenuous activity and to avoid sex for at least a week after the procedure. Since Greg and his wife were eager to become pregnant, the urologist told Greg using an alternative method was not necessary.

Greg followed the urologist's instructions, and his wound healed without difficulty. Three months later, Greg underwent a semen analysis that confirmed that sperm was once again contained within Greg's semen. Greg and his wife began to have sex regularly to increase their chances of becoming pregnant. After several months of trying, Greg's wife finally became pregnant.

Analysis

Men have few options available to participate in contraception. A vasectomy, however, is intended to be a nonreversible form of sterilization for men. Like the female tubal ligation, a vasectomy in males severs an essential tube, or conduit, that sperm requires for transport, so it can mix with semen and seminal fluid. When a man's semen and seminal fluid are lacking sperm, there is no chance an egg can be fertilized by him.

When a vasectomy is performed, each vas deferens is cut, and the two severed ends are typically closed off with sutures, clips, cautery, or a combination of each. A follow-up sperm analysis three months after the procedure confirms the absence of sperm in the semen. Some men, like Greg, may desire to have children years after a successful vasectomy. There is a possibility for a vasectomy to be reversed through a similar surgical procedure.

Many factors impact the success of a vasectomy reversal procedure and future pregnancy for a couple. For example, the more time that has elapsed since the vasectomy was performed, the surgeon's skill, or the age of the female partner trying to conceive can affect whether a vasectomy reversal, overall, will work. Greg's vasectomy was performed less than 10 years ago, and his urologist was experienced at performing the vasectomy reversal procedure. Greg followed the necessary postoperative instructions to promote his healing. The follow-up sperm analysis was necessary to confirm that sperm was again present in Greg's semen. Like other couples, Greg and his wife were advised that pregnancy may or may not occur immediately. However, repeated episodes of unprotected sex with orgasm and ejaculation of semen into the vagina increased Greg's chances of fathering a child, and his wife became pregnant several months after the vasectomy reversal procedure was completed.

Case Study 5: Denise

Denise is a 24-year-old college graduate, who works a full-time job. She has been dating the same man for three years and became pregnant unexpectedly after graduating from college. While Denise was excited about the prospect of motherhood, she had hoped to postpone having children until she became more established in her career and was married. She voiced her feelings to her obstetrician during a routine prenatal visit, and the physician advised Denise that beginning contraception could occur immediately after the baby was born. Denise was given several options that were appropriate for her, including the long-acting, reversible hormonal options such as the contraceptive implant or hormonal injections. The obstetrician thoroughly reviewed the risks and benefits of each, specifically highlighting the potential for menstrual irregularity or the absence of a menstrual period after several months of use and the potential delayed return to fertility once Denise stopped using either method. The obstetrician gave Denise printed material to review and suggested several websites for her to explore for more information.

Denise delivered a baby girl and began breastfeeding. Because Denise intended to exclusively breastfeed her daughter, she opted to use the injectable form of long-acting, reversible hormonal contraception. In addition, Denise planned to wait several years before having another baby, so a method with an uncertain duration for a return to fertility was acceptable to her. Denise received her first injection of depo-medroxyprogesterone (DMPA) at her six-week post-delivery appointment with her obstetrician. Before leaving the appointment, the office staff secured and confirmed Denise's follow-up appointment within 11–12 weeks, so she could return for her next injection.

Following her first injection of DMPA, Denise noticed irregular vaginal bleeding and some unpredictable pink spotting. She opted to use condoms for several days to allow time for the DMPA to begin taking effect. Denise continued to successfully breastfeed her daughter and began to pump and store her breastmilk in anticipation to return to work. Three months after she delivered the baby, Denise returned to work.

Despite having erratic spotting, Denise noticed that the spotting was light and the periods she started having were getting lighter and shorter also. Denise resumed exercising regularly and maintained her healthy diet. Her obstetrician reviewed if any side effects were present each time she returned for a DMPA reinjection. Since no harmful or inconvenient side effects were noted, the obstetrician continued Denise on her DMPA regimen indefinitely.

Analysis

Long-acting, reversible hormonal contraception is a viable option for women who want to postpone pregnancy for an extended, or indefinite, time. Since Denise was working and wanted to postpone having more children for several years, long-acting methods are ideal for her. By choosing DMPA, or "Depo," Denise picked an option that allowed her to continue to breastfeed her daughter, avoid using estrogens, and avoid the inconvenience of remembering to take oral contraceptive pills daily or the necessity to use condoms, a diaphragm, or spermicides each time she had sex.

The DMPA injection provided Denise a consistent dose of hormone daily over 12 weeks. Like most women who initiate DMPA, Denise experienced some menstrual irregularity. However, many women, including Denise, cease having menstrual periods after consistent, prolonged use of DMPA. Denise was diligent about keeping her follow-up appointments for reinjections of DMPA every 11–12 weeks, so her dose of hormone remained consistent and her protection against pregnancy was constant. While women frequently report weight gain when using DMPA, Denise maintaining a healthy diet, and regular exercise allowed her to avoid any unnecessary weight gain.

Women like Denise who use DMPA need to understand that a return to fertility varies after they stop using DMPA. To stop using DMPA, Denise will simply stop getting reinjections of the medication. However, the medication needs to completely clear from Denise's system, which can take several weeks or months. Denise will need to consider this potential delay when she develops her plan for future pregnancies.

Glossary

Abortion: The termination of a pregnancy. An abortion can be *induced*, where a women chooses to end her pregnancy, or *spontaneous*, or a "miscarriage," where a women ceases to be pregnant because she could no longer sustain her pregnancy.

Acne: An inflammation or infection of the sebaceous glands in the skin characterized by pimples, typically on the face.

Amenorrhea: The absence of menstruation, or one or more missed menstrual periods. Women who have missed at least three menstrual periods in a row are considered to have amenorrhea.

Anastomosis: Surgical reconnection or rejoining of two anatomical parts, such as the ends of a fallopian tube during tubal ligation reversal.

Diaphragm: A barrier method of birth control, the diaphragm is a bendable, shallow cup that is typically made of silicone and shaped like a saucer, which, combined with a spermicide, covers the cervix to prevent pregnancy.

Dysmenorrhea: The medical term used to describe painful menstrual cramps that occur immediately before or during a woman's monthly menstrual period.

Ectopic pregnancy: A pregnancy that is not in the uterus. The fertilized egg settles and grows in any location other than the inner lining of the uterus. The large majority (95 percent) of ectopic pregnancies occur in the fallopian tube.

Endometrium: The inner lining of the uterus.

Epididymis: A structure on the upper portion of the testicle where sperm is stored.

Epididymitis: Inflammation of the epididymis.

Estrogen: The primary female sex hormone. It is responsible for the development and regulation of the female reproductive system and secondary sex characteristics.

Fertilization: The union of a human egg and sperm, usually occurring in the ampulla of the fallopian tube.

Fibroids: Also called leiomyomas, uterine fibroids are noncancerous tumors that grow on or around the uterus.

Health-care practitioner: A licensed medical provider who can evaluate, diagnose, and treat various conditions or illnesses. Examples include physicians, nurse practitioners, midwives, or physicians' assistants.

Hematoma: A collection of blood outside of blood vessels. Most commonly, hematomas are caused by an injury to the wall of a blood vessel, prompting blood to seep out of the blood vessel into the surrounding tissues. A hematoma can result from an injury to any type of blood vessel (artery, vein, or small capillary). A hematoma usually describes bleeding that has clotted.

Hydrocele: A fluid-filled sac surrounding a testicle that causes swelling in the scrotum.

Hysterectomy: Surgical removal of a woman's uterus or womb. After a hysterectomy, a woman is no longer able to have menstrual periods and cannot become pregnant. Sometimes the surgery also removes the ovaries and fallopian tubes.

Lactation: Describes the secretion of milk from the mammary glands and the period of time that a mother lactates to feed her young (i.e., breast-feeding or nursing).

Menorrhagia: The medical term for heavy menstrual bleeding.

Menstruation: Also called a menstrual period or the "period," it is normal vaginal bleeding that occurs as part of a woman's monthly cycle. Every month, a woman's body prepares for pregnancy. If no pregnancy occurs, the uterus, or womb, sheds its lining. The menstrual blood is partly blood and partly tissue from inside the uterus. It passes out of the body through the vagina.

Ovulation: The release of eggs from the ovaries, occurring when the ovarian follicles rupture and release the secondary oocyte ovarian cells. After ovulation, during the luteal phase, the egg will be available to be fertilized by sperm.

Pelvic inflammatory disease (PID): An infection of the female reproductive organs. It usually occurs when sexually transmitted bacteria spread from the vagina to the uterus, fallopian tubes, or ovaries.

Perimenopause: Also called menopause transition, it begins several years before menopause. It is the time when the ovaries gradually begin to make less estrogen. It usually starts in a woman's 40s but can start in her 30s or even earlier. Perimenopause lasts up until menopause, the point when the ovaries stop releasing eggs.

Post tubal ligation syndrome (PTLS): PTLS is a cluster of symptoms that include heavy or missed periods, hormonal imbalances, and problems that mimic menopause.

Post vasectomy pain syndrome (PVPS): It is due to nerve damage from the vasectomy procedure that leads to persistent testicular or scrotal pain; also called congestive epididymitis or chronic post vasectomy testicular pain.

Premenstrual dysphoric disorder (PMDD): PMDD is a severe form of premenstrual syndrome (PMS). Like PMS, premenstrual dysphoric disorder follows a predictable, cyclic pattern. Symptoms begin in the late luteal phase of the menstrual cycle (after ovulation) and end shortly after menstruation begins.

Premenstrual syndrome (PMS): PMS involves a variety of physical, mental, and behavioral symptoms tied to a woman's menstrual cycle. PMS symptoms and signs occur during the two weeks before a woman's period starts, known as the luteal phase of the menstrual cycle.

Progesterone: A female steroid sex hormone that is secreted by the corpus luteum to prepare the endometrium for implantation, and later by the placenta during pregnancy, to prevent rejection of the developing embryo or fetus.

Progestin: A synthetic progestogen that has similar effects to those of the natural hormone progesterone.

Prolactin: A hormone secreted by the pituitary gland that enables mammals, usually females, to produce milk.

Prostaglandins: Natural substances that are made by cells of the endometrium and other parts of the body. The prostaglandins made in the uterus cause the uterine muscles to contract and promote shedding of the uterine lining during the monthly menstrual period.

Prostate: The male reproductive gland the produces semen and helps propel semen or seminal fluid out of the body during ejaculation.

Semen: Fluid that is emitted from the male reproductive tract that contains sperm cells, which are capable of fertilizing the female eggs.

Seminal fluid: The part of the semen that is produced by various accessory glands such as the prostate gland and seminal vesicles.

Speculum: A duck-bill-shaped device that doctors use to see inside a hollow part of the body and diagnose or treat disease. One common use of the speculum is for vaginal exams. Gynecologists use it to open the walls of the vagina and examine the vagina and cervix.

Spermatocele: An abnormal cyst that develops in the small, coiled tube located on the upper testicle that collects and transports sperm (epididymis).

Tubal ligation: A type of permanent birth control where the fallopian tubes are cut, tied, or blocked to permanently prevent pregnancy. Tubal ligation prevents an egg from traveling from the ovaries through the fallopian tubes and blocks sperm from traveling up the fallopian tubes to the egg.

Vas deferens: An ejaculatory duct that carries sperm and seminal fluid from the epididymis and into the urethra, so it can be ejaculated from the penis.

Vasectomy: A permanent sterilization procedure for men where the vas deferens is blocked or cut to prevent sperm from mixing with semen or seminal fluid.

Directory of Resources

BOOKS

Hatcher, R. A. (2011). *Contraceptive technology*. 20th edition. Atlanta, GA: Bridging the Gap Communications.

Quinn, P. (2018). *Sexually transmitted diseases: Your questions answered*. Santa Barbara: ABC-CLIO/Greenwood.

WEBSITES

American Association of Women's Health, Obstetric, and Neonatal Nurses (AWHONN)—a national professional nursing association dedicated to advancing science and the health of women and newborns internationally.
https://www.awhonn.org/

American College of Nurse Midwives (ACNM)—the professional organization of nurse midwives and midwives internationally, ACNM believes, promotes, and supports education, research, and advocacy for the care of women across the lifespan.
www.midwife.org

American College of Obstetrics and Gynecology (ACOG)—the premier website for the science of obstetrics, gynecology, and women's

health, this website has a search feature that allows anyone to find information on most topics related to women's health.
https://www.acog.org/

American Pregnancy Association—the American Pregnancy Association is a national health organization committed to promoting reproductive and pregnancy wellness through education, support, advocacy, and community awareness.
www.americanpregnancy.org

Baby Center—BabyCenter, a member of the Johnson & Johnson family of companies, provides parents with trusted information, advice from peers, and support for each stage of their child's development. Products include websites, mobile apps, online communities, e-mail series, social programs, print publications, and public health initiatives.
www.babycenter.com

Cornell Health—health information available from Cornell University on a wide range of topics, including women's health and sexual health.
https://health.cornell.edu

Fibroids Treatment Collective—the Fibroid Treatment Collective is a medical group of fibroid experts dedicated to curing fibroids with minimally invasive therapy.
www.fibroids.com

Go Ask Alice!—a team of Columbia University health promotion specialists, health-care providers, and other health professionals who provide free advice, information, and links to other key women's health websites. Questions can be posted to the website for the team anonymously.
http://goaskalice.columbia.edu/basic-page/all-about-alice

Healthline—provides expert content on health-related topics.
www.healthline.com

Medical News Today—a collection of dedicated information pages about specific conditions or subjects, along with other longer, in-depth articles written by a team of news editors and reviewed by scientific subject matter experts.
https://www.medicalnewstoday.com

NuvaRing—an industry-sponsored website that offers information about all aspects of the NuvaRing.
www.NuvaRing.com

Options for Sexual Health—based out of British Columbia, this organization (known as "Opt") provides sexual and reproductive health care, information, and education from a feminist, pro-choice, sex-positive perspective.
http://optionsforsexualhealth.org

Our Bodies, Ourselves (OBOS)—a nonprofit, public interest organization based in Boston, Massachusetts, that develops and promotes evidence-based information on girls' and women's reproductive health and sexuality. OBOS's publications, website, and blog also address the social, economic, and political conditions that affect health-care access and quality of care.
http://www.ourbodiesourselves.org

Parenting.com—a website with links to content and resources for pregnancy, infertility, baby care, health, wellness, and nutrition.
http://www.parenting.com

Plan B—the most popular brand of the morning after pill currently on the market in the United States, this website offers comprehensive information about emergency contraception and about the Plan B One Dose itself.
http://www.planb.ca

Planned Parenthood—a comprehensive website with reliable, easy-to-understand sexual health information for men and women. Links to additional resources are included along with a directory to locate services in a specific area.
https://plannedparenthood.org

Prenatal Possibilities—a comprehensive website with easy-to-understand information about pregnancy, women's health, and health topics.
www.prenatalpossibilities.com

Very Well Health—a resource for reliable, understandable, and up-to-date health information on medical topics.
www.verywellhealth.com

WebMD—a website with multiple topics related to illness, symptoms, medication, and a special section for pregnancy. Multiple birth control

topics are covered. A newsletter is available with useful health information and updates on a variety of health-related topics.
http://www.webmd.com

Women's Health.gov—a user-friendly resource for understanding the
menstrual cycle with links to other women's health information.
https://www.womenshealth.gov/a-z-topics/menstruation-and-men
strual-cycle

Index

About the Author

Paul Quinn, PhD, is a certified nurse midwife and women's health nurse practitioner with over two decades of acute-care experience in both nursing and midwifery practice within hospitals, clinics, and the private sector. An educator and women's health expert, he received his nursing diploma from Saint Vincent's Hospital School of Nursing, New York City; a bachelor of science in nursing from Pace University, New York City; and a master of science in nursing from the College of Mount St. Vincent, Bronx, New York. Later, he received an Advanced Certificate in Midwifery from the State University of New York-Downstate, Brooklyn, New York, and a doctor of philosophy from the City University of New York. He is the creator of the popular website Prenatal Possibilities (www.prenatalpossibilities.com) to provide health, nutrition, and lifestyle information to women across the lifespan and the author of *Sexually Transmitted Diseases: Your Questions Answered*. His research track involves women's health issues, prenatal health and nutrition, and nursing workforce issues.